Doctored Results

THE SUPPRESSION OF LAETRILE
AT SLOAN-KETTERING INSTITUTE
FOR CANCER RESEARCH

Ralph W. Moss, PhD

Published by
EQUINOX PRESS, INC.
PO Box 1076
Lemont, PA 16851
© 2014 by Ralph W. Moss
All Rights Reserved

All photographs © 2014 by Ralph W. Moss
or are in the public domain

Library of Congress Cataloging-in-Publication Data

Moss, Ralph W.
Doctored results : the suppression of laetrile at Sloan-Kettering Institute for
Cancer Research / Ralph W. Moss, PhD. -- First edition.

Includes bibliographical references.
ISBN 978-1-881025-52-8 (alk. paper)
1. Laetrile. 2. Cancer--Chemotherapy--Research--United States. 3. Drugs-
-Research--Corrupt practices--United States. 4. Pharmaceutical poli-
cy--United States. 5. Memorial Sloan-Kettering Cancer Center. 6. United
States. Food and Drug Administration. I. Title.
RC271.L3M67 2014
616.99'4061--dc23
2013051222

Disclaimer

The information provided in this book is for general educational purposes only. Neither the author nor the publisher makes warranties, expressed or implied, that this information is complete nor do they warrant the fitness of this information for any particular purpose. This information is not intended as medical advice, and they disclaim any liability resulting from its use. Neither the author nor the publisher advocates any treatment modality, including any that are discussed in this book. Each reader is strongly urged to consult qualified professional help for medical problems, including board-certified medical oncologists, when appropriate. Decisions about treatment facilities should be made on the basis of current capabilities, and not on the basis of past deeds or misdeeds.

SKI Paper

In this book, the "final SKI paper on laetrile" refers to "Stock CC, Martin DS, Sugiura K, et al. Antitumor tests of amygdalin in spontaneous animal tumor systems. *Journal of Surgical Oncology.* 1978;10:89–123." When a page number is given in parentheses in the text, it refers to this paper. Readers can obtain a copy at medical libraries, through interlibrary loan, via an institutional online subscription or by paying the publisher, Wiley, $35.00 for personal use, at www.onlinelibrary.wiley.com

Acknowledgements

The author would like to thank the following for commenting on various drafts of this book:

Bharat B. Aggarwal, PhD, Houston, TX; Tibor Bakacs, MD, PhD, DSc, Budapest, Hungary; Keith Block, MD, Skokie, IL; Penny Block, PhD, Skokie, IL; Charlotte Gyllenhaal, PhD, Chicago, IL; Joseph Mahoney, PhD, Reading, PA; Eric Merola, Santa Monica, CA; Peter Pedersen, PhD, Baltimore, MD; Young Ko, PhD, Baltimore, MD; Michael Schachter, MD, Suffern, NY.

Find these books and much more at _The Moss Report_ website.

https://www.themossreport.com/

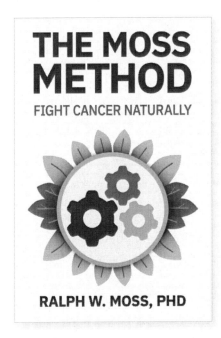

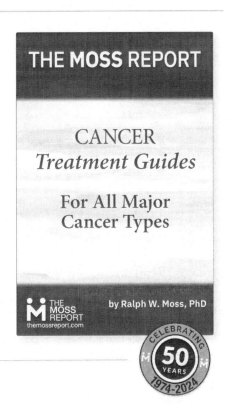

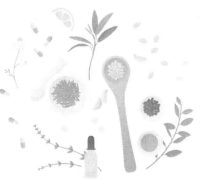

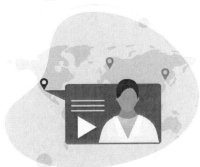

Discover _themossreport.com_ – an indispensable resource offering a wealth of articles, books, videos, podcasts, and natural products to support the fight against cancer.

Explore our site for a unique perspective on integrative oncology around the world.

- _Video Tours of Clinics_
- _Doctor Interviews_
- _Practitioner Map with 1000s of resources... and much more!_

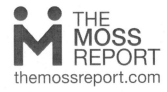

themossreport.com

Contents

Personal History

I began my career as a medical writer in 1974. Like many in my profession, I didn't train to be a researcher, much less to write about scientific advances for the general public. For the previous dozen years, in fact, I had been immersed in the study of ancient civilizations. Then, within a month of receiving my doctorate in Classics from Stanford University, I went to work at Memorial Sloan-Kettering Cancer Center (MSKCC) in New York City writing articles for the public on cancer.

In college my main academic interest was poetry and I went into Classics to read the ancient Greek poets, especially Homer. It was no coincidence that my girlfriend (later my wife), Martha, was already studying ancient Greek at Hunter College. As an undergraduate at Washington Square College of New York University I became excited about the prospects of teaching Classics as a profession.

My mentor at NYU, Prof. Francis E. Peters, gave me the freedom to pursue whatever academic areas interested me most. Earlier in life, he had been a Jesuit seminarian, and although he had given up his priestly career (an evolution he later described in his memoir, *Ours*), he instilled in me an intense interest in some of the topics he had studied in the seminary. Peters' influence on this "nice Jewish boy from Brooklyn" was unexpected, but I derived an indefinable pleasure investigating arcane areas of literary scholarship. Some of these topics, such as "Allegorical Exegesis," remain so obscure that there are still no Wikipedia articles on them.

In my junior year, I also developed an intense interest in the history of Judaism in the Greco-Roman period. I was fascinated by the intersection of Hellenic and Hebrew civilizations and read Flavius Josephus and Philo of Alexandria in Greek. Although my maternal grandfather, Wolf Greenfield, had been Cantor of the Manhattan Beach Jewish Center, I did not come from a religious family. Yet I hired an Israeli graduate student to teach me Biblical Hebrew every Monday night.

In addition to Greek, Latin and a little Hebrew, I learned to read French and German passably well and took courses in Sanskrit and Indo-European.

linguistics. Later, I became one of the few people who could read Oscan and Umbrian inscriptions. At NYU, I also studied philosophy with a famous interpreter of existentialism, Prof. William Barrett (author of *Irrational Man*).

But the high point of my undergraduate career came about as the result of a practical joke. Prof. Peters asked each student in our Greek class to memorize a few lines of Homer's *Iliad*. Carried away by enthusiasm for ancient poetry, and with time to kill while waiting for the uptown subway, I memorized the first 135 lines of the *Iliad* in Greek. (Homer sounds great when echoed off the walls of a nearly empty subway station!) By chance, I was the last person that day whom Peters called upon to recite. When I came to the end of my assigned lines I said, in an offhand way, "Shall I go on?"

Peters nodded yes, and I then fluently recited about 100 lines of Greek epic poetry from memory. At that moment, providentially, the bell rang. The following fall, in his large Near Eastern history class, Peters said, in a deadpan way: "In ancient times it was common for palace watchmen to memorize all 15,693 lines of the *Iliad*. Even today there are rare individuals who know the entire poem by heart. And we happen to have such a person in our class."

He nodded towards me. "Mr. Moss?" he said, with a sly smile. "Would you give us a sample."

I began to recite the pages I had committed to memory. My limits would soon have been discovered, except that Peters had timed the joke perfectly: once again my memorized lines ran out just as the dismissal bell sounded. This spur-of-the-moment joke established my reputation as a kind of "idiot savant" of Homeric poetry at NYU!

Peters, in addition to his mastery of Greek and Latin, had a doctorate from Princeton University in Islamic Studies and later became the founding director of NYU's Hagop Kevorkian Center for Near Eastern Studies. Had I stayed at NYU, I would probably have concentrated on ancient Near Eastern Studies. This might have yielded a very pleasant and productive career indeed.

In May 1964, Martha and I got married and I moved to her apartment on West 75th Street in Manhattan. This was just one room, with the kitchen in a converted closet, but what a room! It had been the billiard parlor of a Victorian mansion built by the publisher, Henry Hobart Vail. It had a Tiffany glass skylight, chestnut shutters and bookshelves, and breathtaking views of the Hudson River. Getting married turned out not to be a financial hardship, either. As soon as he learned that I had gotten married, Dean Philip Mayerson arranged for me to receive a full scholarship for my final year. (It didn't hurt that he was one of my Latin teachers.)

In retrospect, what undid my career in Classics was something happening halfway around the world: the Vietnam War. It was not that I was ever in danger of being drafted. Our daughter Melissa was born in December 1965 and our son Benjamin came along in June 1967, both very providential for my 3-A draft exemption.

But starting with the assassination of President Kennedy in November 1963, our world (along with that of millions of our contemporaries) seemed to veer out of control. There was a series of events that not only dominated the headlines, but led to a roller coaster ride of wrenching emotions: the assassination of Malcolm X, Martin Luther King and Robert Kennedy; the Senate's duplicitous Tonkin Gulf Resolution; and even the massive Northeast blackout of November 1965 and a quickly ensuing transit strike undermined our faith in the government and our hopes for a peaceful future.

One day, towards the end of my senior year, I went to hear the antiwar activist Daniel Berrigan speaking at NYU's Loeb Student Center about his recent "peace mission" to Hanoi. In his lecture, he showed photographs of cluster bombs, napalmed children, and lunar surface devastation caused by the relentless US bombing. These pictures are familiar today, but were indescribably shocking at the time. Like many others, I made an internal pledge to do whatever I could to help stop the slaughter. My reading turned from Allegorical Exegesis to the origins of the Vietnam War.

In 1965, Martha and I attended our first antiwar demonstration. The march was small compared to what was to come and, near the United Nations, we marchers found ourselves tightly fenced in between police barricades. I was shocked when I overheard one booted and helmeted New York City policeman remark to another, "We should march them all into the ovens." He didn't sound like he was kidding.

After graduation in June 1965, I took a job as an Investigator in Harlem for the New York City Department of Welfare. Martha continued to work for the Archaeological Institute of America. Our plan was to work for a year and save up for our 'Grand Tour' of Europe. This was just one year after the Harlem riots, and my job as an Investigator was an eye-opening experience, especially for an erstwhile scholar of Classical poetry. The job went reasonably well until four young men mugged me in broad daylight on West 135th St. I had the nightmarish experience of pedestrians literally stepping over my prone body as my assailants went through my pockets. Finally, some storekeepers, wielding iron pipes, chased them away, but my throat was sore for weeks from my assailants' chokehold. At my supervisor's insistence, I never went out into the field again.

Our daughter, Melissa, was born a few weeks later and in February 1966, in the midst of a blinding snowstorm, our little family of three left for Europe via Icelandic Air (the only airline flying that night). My parents were beside themselves with fright but Martha and I had arguments (nonsensical in retrospect) for why it was perfectly safe for us to take our infant daughter to Europe in the midst of a blizzard. Although our brand new Volkswagen "Bug" and most of our possessions were stolen two weeks later in Marseille we managed to get through this experience in one piece and return to New York in the late spring.

Before leaving for Europe, I had applied to graduate school at Harvard, Yale and Stanford Universities. While I was gone, I received acceptance letters from all three, but only Stanford offered me a full ride—a three-year National Defense Education Act (NDEA) Fellowship. Soon after returning to New York, we undertook an 11-day road trip to California along with Martha's teenage sister, Susan. The four of us crammed into a tiny Fiat 600 with a canvas tent, baby carriage and assorted paraphernalia strapped to the roof.

We camped out every night except the one night we spent in a motel in Chicago. Since neither Martha nor Sue could drive, I handled nearly 4,000 miles by myself. One night, in the desert outside Winnemucca, Nevada, I became so exhausted that I pulled into a rest area, tumbled out of the car and fell asleep right there on the ground! When we finally reached California, I was ticketed for not having a side mirror: Fiat 600s did not come with mirrors then, and I had driven the entire distance without a passenger side mirror. Needless to say, automotives was not my strong suit.

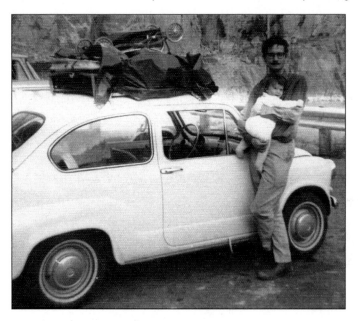

Author with daughter, cross-country trip, 1966

Stanford University in Palo Alto was achingly beautiful. But because of my growing fixation on the Vietnam War, I was in no mood for its country club perfection. We had a very affordable garden apartment in Escondido Village, Stanford's married student housing development, and we enrolled Melissa in the Psychology Department's Bing Nursery School. When Benjamin came along in 1967 Stanford generously upgraded us to a larger apartment. What could be better? But, ironically, the better Stanford treated me, the more alienated I felt.

Recently, the National Research Council ranked Stanford's Classics Department number one in the USA.[2] But in the 1960s, it was beset with problems. There was a sharp division between the junior and senior faculty, who occupied different floors of the department's offices near the Quad. By and large, the older Classics professors could not understand the emotional turmoil of the students or even the younger professors. I later heard that Prof. Lionel Pearson had opposed my entry into the program, referring to me (based on the photo that accompanied my application) as a "bomb thrower." In fact, I have never thrown any bombs, but my shaggy "Greenwich Village" appearance frightened him.

The Stanford Classics Department's idea of pedagogy was quite different than the liberal treatment I had experienced at NYU. At Stanford, the emphasis was on mastering the intricacies of grammar. Here I was at a disadvantage, as I had only started my study of ancient languages in college (not in Prep School or Catholic high school, as had many of my classmates). I particularly dreaded Greek and Latin composition. I would make mistakes and then, to save time, would fix my homework with correction fluid. But my instructor, who was a petty tyrant, would hold my corrected paper up to the light in order to criticize my original mistakes!

One day in 1967, I saw a crowd gathering outside the Hoover Tower. Inquiries revealed that this was a demonstration against CIA recruiters on campus. I realized that, for the sake of my family and my career, I should ignore this protest and get to class. For a moment I even thought I heard my mother's voice telling me to cross the street.

Instead, I made my way to the front line. What had drawn the people was an impromptu debate between two Stanford luminaries. The older man was Bertram D. Wolfe, who had long before turned from American Communist propagandist to ardent anti-Communist and was now a fellow of the conservative Hoover Institution. His antagonist was H. Bruce Franklin, PhD, a charismatic young English professor, a former US Air Force intelligence officer who had returned from a sabbatical year in Paris as a committed Maoist.

Wolfe, author of the classic text, *Three Who Made the Revolution*, taunted Franklin by calling Josef Stalin a thug who robbed banks on behalf of the revolutionary movement. Franklin, with impeccable timing, shot back: "The difference between you and me, Wolfe, is that you think the banks should rob the people, while I think the people should rob the banks."

This got an appreciative laugh from the audience, myself included.

My three years at Stanford (1966-1969) coincided with some of the fiercest fighting of the Vietnam War and the most tumultuous days in the history of the University. Things progressed from rallies to demonstrations to the occupation of University buildings. Demonstrators took over Encina Hall and other campus buildings. Hardly a day went by that there wasn't a protest at White Plaza.

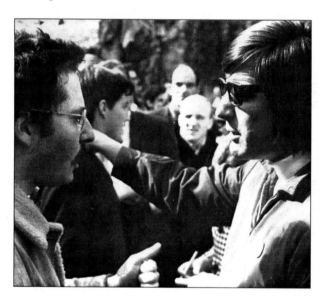

Author, on left, at a demonstration on Stanford campus, 1968

This culminated in the Administration calling outside police onto the campus for the first time in the school's history. The police then tear gassed demonstrators in a wild melee outside the Stanford Research Institute and, on another occasion, in a residential area of Palo Alto adjoining the campus. Residents staggered out of their bungalows, coughing and choking with wet handkerchiefs over their faces.

"It was pretty much a descent into hell," was Provost Richard Lyman's summation, many years later. Students of today, he said, cannot imagine what "a mess" Stanford was in, "with its boarded-up windows, police actions, violence and arson... Even I find it difficult to capture the fears and passions of that turbulent time."[3] However, we demonstrators felt justified in helping to bring about an end to a horrendous war.

I was in a Greek history class in February 1968 when the Tet Offensive broke out in South Vietnam. The National Liberation Front (or "Vietcong") simultaneously attacked hundreds of cities, towns and army bases at a time when our government was assuring us that they were all but defeated. This rolling attack went on for days. Someone brought a portable radio to class and most of us in the back of the room discreetly followed news of the fighting. It was hard to concentrate on ancient Greek sea voyages when world-shaking events were taking place in our own time.

But our visiting professor, a humorless German, wasn't amused and retaliated by giving almost everyone a grade of D. Luckily, our kindly department chairman, Brooks Otis, changed this black mark to a B. I did enjoy my Roman history classes: the violence and turmoil of Roman Republican times seemed to resonate with our own. I managed to finish three years of course work with good grades, although my heart wasn't in it. But the enthusiasm that I had felt for a career in Classics when I was at NYU had largely evaporated.

In the summer of 1969 my three-year NDEA fellowship ran out. Typical of the way I managed my affairs at that time, I hadn't bothered to line up a new position. That would have been too bourgeois! So I took the first temporary job that came along, which was digging ditches in the mud flats of San Francisco Bay. It was as hard as it sounds, but for a while I actually enjoyed this break from Academia.

Our crew operated out of a wooden shack about a mile across the flats from Redwood City; only a single telephone wire, strung on poles, broke the monotony of the muddy plains. As in a movie, suddenly the old-fashioned telephone rang noisily and the call turned out to be for me. Prof. Theodore "Ted" Brunner, a Stanford alumnus who ran the Classics Department at the University of California, Irvine, was looking for a young instructor and Prof. Otis had kindly suggested me. After a whirlwind visit to Orange County, with lunch at a riverboat restaurant and a tour of the Gold Coast, I checked with Martha and then accepted a two-year contract. I hoped that a new venue, together with serious teaching responsibilities, might rekindle my interest in Classics as a profession.

And so, after three years in a troubled paradise, Martha, Melissa, Benjamin and I packed our possessions in our red-and-white VW van and set off for new adventures in Southern California.

From my description, Martha pictured a land of orange blossoms. Well, that was the way Newport Beach and Laguna Beach looked to me on my whirlwind tour. But a few miles in the interior we found a bleak landscape, with many of the orange trees radically uprooted to make way for a university-based metropolis on Joan Irvine's 100,000-acre ranch. Martha actually started crying and told me to "turn left," meaning to head back to New York. But I explained that I had signed a contract and was obligated to stay.

I was no less discontented in my office trailer on the edge of campus than I had been at Stanford. UC Irvine today is quite verdant. But the school had just opened its doors in 1965 and even in the late 1960's was so barren that Hollywood producers chose it as the setting for a dystopic movie, *Conquest of the Planet of the Apes*.

I was supposed to be finishing my doctoral dissertation but hadn't even decided on a topic. Again, politics took priority. This was the era of the wanton shooting of students at Kent State and Jackson State (May 1970), which quickly led to the shutdown of hundreds of college campuses across the country. Martha and I were in the thick of the protests on the Irvine campus. After the shootings, I put it up to my students whether or not to even hold classes. They decided to spend class time discussing world events (although some were understandably furious at this decision).

One memorable confrontation was with the chancellor of the university, Daniel C. Aldrich, PhD. Aldrich was trying to explain why he refused to shut down the University in the wake of the killings. At one point he said, "We've got to separate the wheat from the chaff."

One of the student protesters responded in frustration, "It's all bullshit!" Without missing a beat, Aldrich—himself a farmer and soil chemist—replied, "You're right, it is all bullshit. But we've got to separate the wheat from the chaff *in* the bullshit."

This drew a laugh from the demonstrators and helped defuse tensions. That witty saying has come in handy for me in life on many occasions.

One unexpected development was that I found myself gravitating towards the history of science. Perhaps at the time science, even ancient science, seemed more "relevant" than literature. Ted Brunner and his colleagues generously allowed me to teach a course on Hippocratic Medicine in Greek, which I enjoyed. I also began to incorporate extended discussions of ancient science and technology into my civilization courses. (I continued to do so at Hunter College.) But I still felt alienated from the typical Classics curriculum and from academic life in general.

We left Irvine when my contract ended in May 1971. From 1971 to 1973 I worked on my dissertation in a desultory way, while holding various odd jobs around the Los Angeles area. It was a generally bleak time and we moved often. The most memorable event was a 1971 earthquake, measuring six on the Richter scale, which literally knocked our kids out of their beds and left a jagged crack straight through our rental house.

In the spring of 1973 we decided to go back East, almost seven years since the start of our California adventure. Since leaving without an advanced degree would have felt like a huge failure, I approached Stanford and asked for an appointment to take my oral exams. They did not seem surprised either by my four-year absence or my sudden reappearance. It turned out that of my 18 classmates who had started in the Classics graduate program in 1966 only two had actually obtained their PhDs. I aimed to be the third.

I studied hard for a few months, mainly by jumping from article to article in the *Oxford Classical Dictionary*. I then flew to Stanford and passed my orals. My two areas of specialization were Homer's *Odyssey* and ancient slavery. In the meantime, my dissertation advisor, Brooks Otis, had left Stanford for the University of North Carolina, Chapel Hill, and so there was a practical reason for me to return East as well.

We drove back to New York, our third cross-country trip. Melissa was now eight and Ben six. It was not easy crossing the country with two kids in the back of our rickety VW van. We had set up a kind of handmade bunk bed in the rear, the kind that would never pass inspection today—two kids playing in, around and on top of a wooden structure as the car barreled along the Interstate highways at its top speed of 75 mph. One time, in Missouri, the car hydroplaned on a slick stretch of the Interstate and wound up hurtling down an embankment, luckily not a steep one. A kindly family in a station wagon passed us, screeched to a halt, and came running back with cups of apple juice for all of us.

"It's going to be white knuckles all the way," said our Good Samaritan. And he was right. Late one night, after fleeing a bed-buggy motel in Pennsylvania, we finally crossed the Verrazzano-Narrows Bridge. I pulled the car over to the side of the road, got out and literally kissed the good earth of Brooklyn.

Over the next year I finished my dissertation while teaching Classics at Hunter College of the City University of New York. The Department chair there was Prof. Clairève Grandjouan, who had been Martha's boss at the Archaeological Institute of America. (Tragically, Clairève died of breast cancer a few years later.)

However, 1974 was a recession year, and all Clairève could offer me was a half-time appointment. Therefore, to earn extra money, I worked at the Third Avenue public relations firm of Monica de Hellerman. My most memorable client was a man who billed himself the "Coconut King." I became an instant expert on many unexpected uses of the coconut.

Martha, who has had a remarkable variety of jobs in her life, found work as a medical editor for *Urology Times*. We were happy to be back in New York City, especially since both our families were nearby. But, needless to say, this was nothing like what I had imagined life would be like when I was a student a decade before at New York University.

The Vietnam War was winding down, as was the urgency of my belief in various social causes. At the same time, the "War on Cancer" was starting to excite everyone's imagination. President Nixon had officially declared this new "war" on December 23, 1971. Aides called this his "Christmas Present to the Nation."[4] In 1974 the effort was still almost brand new, but it seemed as if, finally, a cure for cancer was at hand. At the time there were very few large cancer hospitals, and Memorial Sloan-Kettering Cancer Center (MSKCC), due east of Hunter College, was the largest and the greatest. Most people figured that the most important discoveries would inevitably come from there.

Our friends all knew that we needed more income for our young family. A colleague at Hunter heard that a job was opening at MSKCC for a science writer. Since she knew of my wife's work at *Urology Times*, she suggested that Martha apply. When I called Martha to tell her about the job opening, she made the outlandish suggestion that I apply for it myself. I was startled. But, after much discussion, I agreed to apply for it. I had my interest in the history of science, plus I figured that medical terminology would not be a problem because most of it was barely disguised Latin and Greek. I was still looking for something more "relevant" than Classics, and what could be more meaningful than helping publicize a cure for cancer?

Although I had no experience in writing about science, I knew that I could do the job if I set my mind to it. With trepidation, in early March 1974 I called for an appointment. I was happily surprised when the secretary of the Director of Public Affairs called me back to set up an interview. What had begun as a long shot was now turning serious.

Memorial Sloan-Kettering Cancer Center was in the process of completing its move to a new hospital building on York Avenue between 67th and 68th Streets. I quickly learned that MSKCC was the parent corporation of two world famous organizations: Memorial Hospital for Cancer and Allied Diseases, which was founded in 1884, and the Sloan-Kettering Institute for Cancer Research, which was organized in 1945. While the patient floors of the new hospital were already open, some ancillary departments, such as Public Affairs, had not yet moved in. Public Affairs (which is a fancy name for public relations) was temporarily housed in a warehouse-like building on East 62nd Street. The head of the department was T. Gerald "Jerry" Delaney, a boyish-looking man in his early forties.

Jerry was born in 1931 in Lincoln, Nebraska but grew up in the small town of Polson Lake, Montana, where his father was an attorney in private practice. Jerry came East for his college education at Georgetown University. His clean-cut good looks reminded me of the former mayor of New York, John Lindsay. Jerry's most memorable trait was that he blushed easily (which, for an employee, made him quite easy to "read").

In those days there were few academic programs devoted to educating medical writers, who were consequently recruited from diverse fields. My pitch to Sloan-Kettering was the same as an early science writer, Gerard Piel, had used to get his first job at *Life* magazine. Piel had been a history major at Harvard but had convinced the publisher Henry Luce to hire him because he was, as he later put it, "certifiably illiterate in science." Piel went on to become the legendary publisher of *Scientific American*. He recalled:

> "The idea was that if I could understand what I was writing
> and publishing, then so could the reader. I became a science
> journalist and my education has been continuing ever
> since."[5]

That was the same tack that I used to get hired at MSKCC: I was a *tabula rasa*, a blank slate, upon which they could write their story. I knew I was a long shot for the job, but my doctorate was a big plus in my favor. Jerry liked the idea of improving the tone of the department by employing a writer with a PhD after his name. Plus I was willing to work for $13,500, which was relatively little even at that time.

I had intellectual curiosity and enthusiasm, and I wanted the job badly. But because of my unconventional background, Jerry hesitated before hiring me. The previous writer had left suddenly and they needed contributors to *Center News*, so Jerry was willing to try me out on a free-lance basis. I had to go through a series of "tests," which lasted several months.

Jerry handed me scientific articles from one of Sloan-Kettering's founding members, Aaron Bendich, PhD (1917-1979).[6] Among other things, Bendich had shown that sperm could penetrate not just eggs but normal body cells and then insert its DNA into the nuclei of these recipient cells.[7] (Subsequent research has shown that sperm do enter somatic cells relatively easily, but that "mechanisms exist to eliminate sperm-derived" DNA from these cells.[8])

Armed with reprints of Bendich's papers, and a fresh copy of *Stedman's Medical Dictionary*, I typed my first science article on the dining room table of our tiny apartment on Ocean Avenue, while our normal family life went on around me. I then held my breath. Jerry liked it, as did Dr. Bendich. A month before I was formally hired, my first article appeared in *Center News*.

The other part of the hiring process was to be interviewed by an array of top officials of the Center. The first was Mr. Charles Forbes, vice president for Development and Public Affairs. "Charlie" Forbes was a soft-spoken and beautifully tailored Southerner, a fundraiser who kept copies of the *Social Register* prominently displayed on his bookshelf.

I then met with Edward "Ted" Beattie, MD, the head of the hospital, an affable man, and with Robert A. "Bob" Good, MD, PhD, head of the Institute. Good was well known from the recent cover story on him in *Time* magazine. He had a larger-than-life personality and actually seemed interested in me. I remember we discussed the differences between research in the Humanities and the Sciences. I also met briefly with Lewis Thomas, MD, President of MSKCC who was, in a sense, Beattie and Good's "boss." (In actuality, he was chief among equals.)

At Jerry's suggestion I looked up Thomas' essays, which were then appearing in the *New England Journal of Medicine,* and were creating a sensation. They were eventually collected into a thin volume, *Lives of a Cell,* which won the National Book Award in 1975. Like much of America, I was enchanted by these charming and humane articles and intended to model my own writing on his. But my initial meeting with Thomas was disappointing. He sat in his sky-high office on the 21st floor of the hospital, puffing on his pipe, and saying as little as possible. Compared to him, Alice's Caterpillar was a chatterbox.

In May 1974, I was informed that I had gotten the job of full-' science writer in the Department of Public Affairs. The weel' starting, Martha and I celebrated our tenth wedding anniversa' a rare vacation. As we sat on the porch of a B&B in Cape C' plated our future. We knew the changes would be h' excited by the opportunity. Finally, I had obtained a job that seemed worthy of my energy and enthusiasm. But, of course, neither of us had any idea of the strange direction in which fate would quickly lead us.

When I took up my new position, on June 3, 1974, Jerry took me on an introductory tour to meet my coworkers. I was then assigned a tall, windowless space, more like a storage room than an office. It would be a year before I could exchange it for a nice office on the 20th floor of the new hospital.

Jerry handed me a manila folder bulging with letters from the public that were long overdue in answering. On the front, in block letters, someone had written the word "PSHAW." I assumed that "PSHAW" was a genteel exclamation of contempt, impatience or disgust. But it turned out to be the first initial and last name of my predecessor, Phyllis Shaw.

In that pre-Internet era, these letters—painstakingly typed or handwritten—were the public's way of connecting with the war on cancer, as well as a way of sharing personal problems. There were inquiries about specific therapies, suggestions concerning possible treatments, and, occasionally, the ramblings of a paranoid schizophrenic. For example, one elderly lady in Maine believed that the cure for cancer could be found in the subterranean waters that flowed under the evergreen trees on her property. I naively called around to see if anyone was willing to test this water, but nobody was. In fact most scientists seemed bemused by the request.

This was the backlog of Phyllis's job, which nobody else in the department wanted to deal with. So, naturally, the job fell to the new guy.

Many of the "PSHAW letters" concerned a substance called amygdalin, or, more popularly, laetrile. This was a treatment derived from the kernel of the apricot pit, which to judge from these letters had wonderful qualities against cancer. I had heard of this once before: on Sunday, March 31, 1974, with 20 million other Americans, I had listened as Mike Wallace (on *60 Minutes*) described how Americans were traveling to Mexico to get this unapproved cancer treatment. There was even a brief mention of experiments at Sloan-Kettering, but at that moment I became distracted by some minor family emergency and didn't pay any special attention to the TV. The takeaway message, I gathered, was that desperate people would do just about anything to find a cure. It was surely just another example of the madness and delusion of crowds.

As I read through the PSHAW letters, I realized that some people were angry, very angry that MSKCC wasn't properly testing laetrile or refused to use this apricot pit "cure." To answer them, Jerry gave me a carefully worded statement that had been drawn up a year before. It said that the testing of laetrile at Sloan-Kettering Institute was ongoing but that, to date, it had been found to have no effectiveness in treating or preventing cancer. People should not abandon their proven, conventional treatments. The prevailing attitude in our office towards laetrile was one of mild amusement or skeptical disbelief.

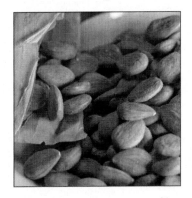

Apricot kernels, source of laetrile

My duties as MSKCC's science writer were hardly onerous. I had to contribute a three-page news article to *Center News* every month, plus an occasional longer feature piece. I periodically wrote press releases and contributed the research section of MSKCC's *Annual Report*. But I had the freedom to interview whichever scientists I chose, in their laboratories. Nothing could have been more fascinating. I felt as if I were getting a top-notch introduction to science and was getting paid for it, to boot! Sloan-Kettering was my "Yale College and my Harvard" (to quote Melville on the topic of whaling ships).

My boss, Jerry Delaney, had a boyish appetite for science, the more "gee whiz" the better. So, in addition to my written job description, I became his personal interpreter of new research (although I hardly knew more than he did). By doing this, I got good practice in talking about complicated subjects in a way that was intelligible to the general public. I had an almost endless supply of fascinating people to talk to and learn from. In short, I couldn't have been happier with my new job.

The War on Cancer

The US government had had an organized cancer research program since passage of the National Cancer Institute (NCI) Act of 1937. But by the late 1960s, cancer was killing almost 350,000 Americans per year. (The current figure is 580,000.) This program had already accomplished many important things, including the identification of tobacco as the major cause of lung cancer. There was a thriving program in identifying environmental and industrial causes of cancer. But in certain quarters there was a general feeling that the NCI had not made sufficient progress in finding a cure for the disease.

The astonishing success of the Atomic Bomb project, the polio vaccine and the race to the moon had put many Americans in an optimistic mood.[10] Many believed that if sufficient resources were directed towards the goal, a concerted effort could find a cure. A secondary advantage would be to help close the Cold War "science gap" that had opened with the Russians' successful launch of the Sputnik satellite in 1957.

Towards this end, in 1970, the US Senate appointed a blue-ribbon National Panel of Consultants on the Conquest of Cancer, whose purpose, according to its chairman, Ralph Yarborough (D-Tex.), was:

> *"To recommend to Congress and to the American people what must be done to achieve cures for the major forms of cancer by 1976...."*[11]

The committee had 26 members, half of whom were laymen. Members included three from MSKCC: its influential board chairman, Laurance S. Rockefeller, its board vice chairman, Benno Schmidt and a Sloan-Kettering Institute (SKI) chemotherapist, Joseph Burchenal, MD.

July 4, 1976 was chosen as the target date because it was to be America's Bicentennial. What a glorious event it would be if our political and medical leaders could announce the cure for cancer on America's 200th birthday! In the foreword to the Consultants' final report, Sen. Yarborough put the case for an all-out assault on cancer:

> *"Cancer is a disease which can be conquered. Our advances*
> *in the field of cancer research have brought us to the verge of*
> *important and exciting developments in the early detection*
> *and control of this dread disease...."[12]*

Sidney Farber, MD, of Boston, one of the pioneers of chemotherapy, was also one of the "prime architects" of the Consultants' report.[13] The "advances" to which Senator Yarborough alluded consisted of toxic drugs that were starting to show a real possibility of curing acute pediatric leukemia. R. Lee Clark, MD, president of the University of Texas M.D. Anderson Cancer Center, Houston, cut to the bottom line:

> *"With a billion dollars a year for ten years we could lick*
> *cancer."[14]*

In the 1960s, America had spent $26 billion to land men on the moon, and the only tangible reward had been a collection of rocks and dust of interest to a few astronomers. At that same time, all of the cancer scientists in the US worked on a budget of $250 million a year—less than one percent of the moon shot's total.[15]

It was a liberal Democrat, Sen. Ted Kennedy (D-MA), who first proposed legislation to expand cancer research by amending the Public Health Service Act. But in that bipartisan era, Republicans took up the cause and on December 23, 1971, President Nixon signed the National Cancer Act, launching a well-funded, full-scale attack on the "Dread Disease."[16]

Adopting the language of the Consultants' report, Congress designated the Act "a national crusade to be accomplished by 1976 in commemoration of the 200th anniversary of our country...." Pres. Nixon in his State of the Union Message called for "the same kind of concentrated effort that split the atom and took man to the moon."

The "War on Cancer" may have expressed a deep desire but only a few people understood that the science was not mature enough to make specific promises. The *Wall Street Journal's* science writer Jerry E. Bishop revealed the illusion at its core:

> *"It is highly unlikely that any group of experts can promise*
> *that cures for major forms of cancer will be achieved within*

*five years even if appropriations for cancer research were
unlimited. To do so [i.e., to make such claims] could raise
high hopes among the public and result in disenchantment,
as 1976 rolled around, that might do considerable harm to
public support of cancer research in the long run. Yet
without such dramatic promises, public enthusiasm for a
major 'assault' on cancer that the researchers have longed for
may be more difficult to arouse.*"[17]

An underlying premise of the National Cancer Act was that the search for a cure had become bogged down in scientific red tape. What was needed, it was thought, was strong leadership, unencumbered by the niceties of protocol. The National Cancer Act removed the budget of the NCI from the control of the National Institutes of Health (NIH), which was considered too bureaucratic to act expeditiously. Congress also approved the creation of a three-member President's Cancer Panel, to advise the President on how to speed progress in the war. The head of this three-member panel was Benno C. Schmidt, Sr., popularly dubbed the "Cancer Czar." This influential layman was supposed to direct attention and dispatch funds to the most important projects. By doing so, the Cure could be found within a few short years.

As it turned out, of course, July 4, 1976 came and went without much notice of the NCI's failure to deliver. At the *Journal of the National Cancer Institute* that July the missed target date went completely unmentioned. In fact, once the "war on cancer" was launched, its continued funding rarely became an issue. Only on milestone anniversaries did an occasional critic surface to wonder about the lack of progress. For instance, Prof. Samuel S. Epstein of the University of Illinois and I wrote two op-eds on the 20th anniversary: "Have We Lost the War on Cancer?" in the *Chicago Tribune*, (December 12, 1991) and "Losing the Cancer War" in *USA Today*, (December 23, 1991). The "war" became institutionalized and NCI funding now totals over $5 billion per year.[18] It seems politically sacrosanct.

The "Cancer Czar" Benno Charles Schmidt, Sr. (1913-1999) was a busy, productive and wealthy man. His "day job" was as managing partner of the J. H. Whitney investment firm. He was also a lawyer, a corporation director and venture capitalist (it is said that he coined the term). Schmidt was not born to wealth. His father had been a traveling salesman who died when he was 12, and the Schmidt family survived on his mother's earnings as a secretary.[19] His big break came when the financier John Hay "Jock" Whitney chose him as his right-hand man.

After becoming national "Cancer Czar," Schmidt retained his position as vice chairman of Memorial Sloan-Kettering Cancer Center's Board of Overseers. The two other President's Cancer Panel members were Robert A. Good, MD, PhD, the newly appointed President of Sloan-Kettering Institute, and R. Lee Clark, MD, president of M.D. Anderson Cancer Center.

Today, the President's Cancer Panel has lapsed into obscurity. But, for a while, it was uniquely influential, and during that time, Sloan-Kettering's influence was unprecedented. Two of the three members on the Panel were Sloan-Kettering leaders, with direct access to the President of the United States.

Schmidt prided himself on his no-nonsense ability to assess the accuracy of scientific claims. I sat in on a few meetings over which he presided and can report that he had a commanding presence, with caterpillar-like eyebrows whose elevation could make underlings shiver.[20]

The long-simmering laetrile problem, which had been roiling the medical scene since 1953, immediately fell in Schmidt's lap. In 1973, President Nixon, his wife, Pat, and all members of Congress received copies of a petition signed by 43,000 Americans. The petitioners demanded that clinical testing of laetrile "start now." The President was relieved that he could refer this hot potato to his "Cancer Czar."[21]

"Since I've been chairman of the President's cancer panel," Schmidt told *Science* magazine in 1973,

> *"I've had literally hundreds of letters about laetrile. Some people ask me whether it is any good. Others flatly state that it cures. A great many say that, in any case, it alleviates pain. When I answer these people and tell them that laetrile has no effect, I would like to be able to do so with some conviction."*[22]

Leaving aside his rather negative way of stating the problem, I believe Schmidt's heart was in the right place. He was eager to do his momentous job right and to turn over every stone, no matter how skeptical his scientific colleagues were about what they considered the most blatant form of cancer quackery.

Schmidt was a layman, and yet this did not preclude his being able to seriously question scientists. In fact, his outsider status was an asset. He began by asking sharp questions, just as he did when he invested "Jock" Whitney's or his own money in a science-based company. Leaders of the National Cancer Institute (NCI) and the American Cancer Society (ACS) gave him vague reassurances that laetrile had been adequately tested and found worthless. But these platitudes did not satisfy him and certainly would not have satisfied the 43,000 angry petitioners. When Schmidt demanded a greater degree of certainty, he recalled, "I couldn't get anybody to show me his work."[23]

The anti-laetrilists, of whom there were many, trotted out a 1953 report from the California Cancer Commission, which was filled with many errors, omissions and inconsistencies. There were also many negative tests in transplantable animal tumor systems, but scientists were gradually losing faith in such artificial systems.

Many people, Schmidt discovered, had opinions about laetrile but few had credible data. Even the journal *Science* (generally skeptical about "alternative" cancer treatments) agreed that prior research into laetrile by "so-called reputable scientists" had been minimal.[24]

What if competent scientists, Schmidt wondered, were to put aside their prejudices against "quackery" and study laetrile in a dispassionate way? What might they find? These seemed like simple enough questions, but it would prove extremely difficult to overcome the prejudices even of notable scientists. Many of them had spoken out emphatically against laetrile in the past and it would prove deeply embarrassing for them to publicly change their minds.

Three Leaders

The Institute that Schmidt turned to for answers was itself in the midst of a major upheaval. Two noted industrialists, Alfred P. Sloan and Charles Kettering, had founded the Sloan-Kettering Institute for Cancer Research in 1945. Both were top executives of General Motors and their approach to finding a cancer cure bore a strong resemblance to the mass production methods of a GM factory.

In 1947, C. Chester Stock, PhD, then at the Rockefeller Institute, was put in charge of testing tens of thousands of compounds in an empirical search for a cancer cure. The thinking was that if enough chemicals were run through a standard panel of tests a cure would inevitably be found.

In a 1963 paper, Stock reported on the screening of drugs in sarcoma 180, a commonly used experimental model. He wrote:

> "Since 1947, when our program began, approximately 25,000 compounds have been screened for ability to inhibit the growth of sarcoma 180...Additionally, since 1950, 40,000 materials of biological origin have been tested."[25]

In other words, Stock had supervised the same procedure 65,000 times in 16 years, 4,000 times per year, or about 25 times each and every working day! The results showed marked inhibition of tumors by just 14 compounds, a "success rate" of 0.0002 percent. Ultimately, not one of these 14 chemicals made it into clinical practice. Dissatisfied with the conspicuous lack of success, and the lack of a theoretical basis for the search, the top leaders of MSKCC, primarily Laurance Rockefeller and Benno Schmidt, decided to shake things up.

In quick succession, they hired Lewis Thomas, MD, to head MSKCC and Robert A. Good, MD, PhD, to head SKI. Good then promoted SKI's most brilliant immunologist, Lloyd J. Old, MD, to be his deputy director. Stock was kept on as the other deputy director, but was in a sense exiled to the institute's Walker research facility in suburban Rye, NY.

In the early 1970s, when the laetrile question arrived at Sloan-Kettering, the three dominant scientific figures were Lloyd J. Old, Robert A. Good and Lewis Thomas. As such, they determined the ultimate fate of laetrile at Sloan-Kettering. We therefore need to know more about each of these leaders.

Lloyd J. Old, MD

In the summer of 1972, Benno Schmidt approached Lloyd J. Old, MD, the wunderkind of immunology, to oversee SKI's testing of laetrile. Old was the perfect choice, as he had a well-deserved "reputation for doing good science without bias" (to quote *Science*[26]). He was youthful, brilliant and open-minded, in an organization that had its share of conformists. That is why Benno Schmidt, himself an unconventional thinker, turned to him for this highly unconventional job.

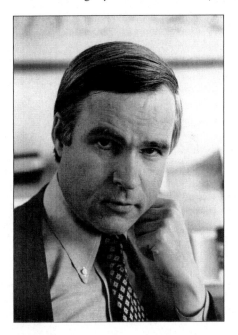

Lloyd J. Old, MD, circa 1975

Lloyd John Old was born in San Francisco on September 23, 1933. His family moved to nearby Burlingame, where he attended the public schools.

He was concertmaster of his high school orchestra, and upon graduation, in 1951, went to Paris for a year to study the violin with European masters.[27]

Multi-faceted, upon his return, he attended the University of California, Berkeley for his Bachelor's degree in biology, and then the University of California, San Francisco (UCSF) for medical school. After driving across the country in a brand new red Corvette, in the summer of 1958 he went to work in the Division of Experimental Chemotherapy at Sloan-Kettering Institute.[28] Old was an imaginative researcher, meticulous writer and loyal team leader, who worked with the same dozen or so individuals for the better part of half a century.

Soon after arriving in New York City, he met a Park Avenue lady who would have a profound effect on his career. She was a banker's wife named Helen Coley Nauts. Helen was the daughter of Memorial Hospital's former bone specialist, William Bradley Coley, MD, who in the 1890s had invented an unorthodox "fever therapy" treatment for cancer.

Helen and Lloyd took to each other and formed a powerful bond, but in a sense they were an odd couple. Lloyd may have had a naturally aristocratic manner, but his father was a German-speaking laborer. Helen was outspoken to the point of asperity, but her genteel family had arrived in America just after the Pilgrims had landed on Plymouth Rock.[29]

Her father, in addition to being one of the top bone specialists in the US, was a director of Memorial Hospital and had been honored for his innovative work on cancer all over the world. When he died in 1936 his son Bradley continued his work both as Memorial Hospital surgeon, author (*Neoplasms of Bone*) and pioneer of the immune therapy of cancer. But, along the way, the Coleys incurred the displeasure of top MSKCC officials, such as Cornelius P. "Dusty" Rhoads, who were thoroughly enamored of chemotherapy.

After the Food and Drug Administration (FDA) refused to "grandfather" Coley's Toxins as an old drug in 1963, its fate was sealed and its use was barred, even at Memorial. Then, in 1965, the American Cancer Society declared Coley's toxins to be an "unproven method of cancer management," the worst thing it could say about any treatment, and Coley descended from pioneering oncologist to habitué of the world's most notorious quack list.

But the ACS didn't reckon with Mrs. Nauts, who embarked on a one-woman crusade to vindicate her father's work and restore her family's good name. With Lloyd Old's help, she wrote a series of scientific monographs showing that her father had cured some 'incurable' cases of cancer with his mixed bacterial vaccine. Through her Park Avenue connections, she successfully raised money for immunology research, first and foremost for Lloyd Old's laboratory. Thus began a unique lifelong partnership.

Together, Lloyd and Helen turned CRI into a scientifically credible organization. In 1971, Lloyd became its Scientific Advisory Council director, a position he held for the rest of his life. Although he also held leadership positions at Sloan-Kettering and the wealthy Ludwig Foundation, CRI remained his intellectual and spiritual home.

Lloyd's scientific achievements over the years were legendary:[30,31]

- He introduced the concept of using Bacillus Calmette-Guérin (BCG) as immunotherapy for cancer.[32]

- He discovered the link between the major histocompatibility complex and a disease, namely leukemia.

- He discovered the association between Epstein-Barr virus and nasopharyngeal carcinoma.

- He and his team discovered tumor necrosis factor.

- He defined the concept of cell-surface differentiation antigens.

- He discovered CD8, otherwise known as "killer T cells."

- He discovered the tumor suppressor p53.

- He identified the tumor immunogenicity of heat shock proteins.

Old was the author or co-author of more than 700 research publications. Any one of his major discoveries would be considered an outstanding lifetime achievement for another individual. He did the work of half a dozen brilliant scientists and had a unique ability to think deeply about numerous problems in immunology, and to see those ideas through to fulfillment.

Old also turned his attention to many alternative treatments, eventually including laetrile. His interest in laetrile actually predated Benno Schmidt's request that he oversee its testing at SKI. Out of scientific curiosity, he had already begun to look at this compound in the spring of 1972.

Old had been profoundly impressed by Coley's story. He was therefore serious about reexamining controversial ideas, regardless of the disapproval of the medical establishment or, for that matter, his MSKCC colleagues. At the start, in my opinion, he was also a bit naïve. He did not yet realize the full extent of opposition to unconventional treatments or that when powerful leaders denounced something as quackery, it was very difficult to contradict them, even if one came armed with new facts.

Meetings with Old

My meetings with Lloyd Old were among the most memorable of my life. For my first year at MSKCC, I could not get to see him, as he seemed to have an aversion to the field of public relations. However, after I wrote an admiring article for *Center News* about Coley, and visited Mrs. Nauts at her Park Avenue apartment, Old indicated that I was welcome to visit him as well.

I therefore went to see him at his office on the 13th floor of the Howard Building. The "art" in most scientists' work spaces consists of *Dilbert* or *Far Side* cartoons taped to the lab refrigerator. But on entering Lloyd Old's salon-like office one saw a beautifully framed oil painting of Wolfgang Amadeus Mozart! As I indicated, he had started out as a violinist and music was his "road not taken." (Many years later, he formed a friendship with members of the Shanghai String Quartet, who played at his 75th birthday party and his memorial service.)

Lloyd Old was a strikingly good-looking man. He proved both brilliant and personable. But he was most comfortable speaking persuasively behind closed doors and was not one to publicly confront people. He was also one of those charismatic leaders who made you feel that you were, however momentarily, the most important person in his life.

Old and I had long talks about many things, including Coley, whose work remained his life-long inspiration. His deep understanding of the Coley saga gave him a natural inclination towards alternative treatments.

Old explained to me that cancer immunotherapy, his chosen field, had originated with the work of Coley. He and his friend Edward "Ted" Boyse, wrote favorably about Coley in their memorable 1973 *Harvey Lecture.*[33] But the testing of Coley's toxins *per se* had stalled. The main effort was to understand the underlying mechanisms of immunity. I asked Old why one couldn't study Coley's toxins themselves, or at least fever therapy, instead of searching for complicated and synthetic substitutes. He voiced the opinion that modern people no longer experienced high fevers the way they had in Coley's day. Perhaps, he said, we had been subjected to too many antibiotics in the food supply to be able any longer to mount a vigorous immune response. Coley's toxins were also difficult to administer and tolerate and thus there was a big compliance issue.

Old was a bit enigmatic even to his friends. "Lloyd was a private person, and I would venture to claim that very few—if any—had the chance to know all of his intricately carved facets," wrote one eulogist, Ellen Puré of the Wistar Institute, Philadelphia, after his death in 2012. "But behind his reserved demeanor, Lloyd was a passionate and very caring man."[34]

Old had his own laboratory, of course, but also had higher ambitions. One could say that he wanted to be "concertmaster" in the cancer research orchestra. Although still quite young, he had waited more than a decade to influence the direction of research at SKI. Now, in 1972, his moment had come when Robert A. Good chose him to be his deputy director.

Fundamentally, then, Lloyd Old was an agent of change, who wanted to move oncology away from the 'slash-burn-and-poison' era into a new age, in which the patient's innate immune system would be harnessed to destroy the disease.

After my first interview, Old and I became friendly. In the spring of 1975, he and Helen Coley Nauts invited me to attend a gala being organized by the Cancer Research Institute at the Hotel Pierre on Fifth Avenue in Manhattan to mark the recognition of immunotherapy (and, by extension, CRI) as an important new force in the cancer field. It would turn out to be a historic occasion.

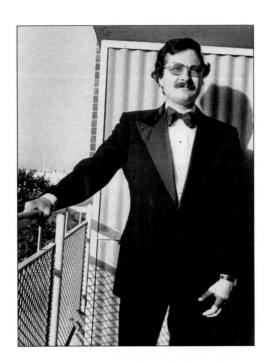

The author on his balcony before the Pierre gala, 1975

Officially, I attended the gala as a reporter from *Center News*. In one of our meetings, Old had said to me, "This will be good for you," meaning it will introduce you to New York society. I didn't consider myself unsophisticated, but this was in fact the first time that I had worn even a rented tuxedo.

I felt a bit uncomfortable in this five star hotel's ballroom, but I soon found another outsider to talk to. This was Lloyd's father, John Hans Old (1904-1980). He was of Swiss and German origin and had come to the US in 1920 to work as a bricklayer and then as a yardman for an oil company. The previous October (1974) he had lost his wife, Edna, Lloyd's mother, to cancer. His sadness was evident.

The highlight of this Pierre Hotel gala was the presentation of the "Founders of Cancer Immunology" awards to 16 scientists, including Good and Old himself. (This is now the annual William B. Coley Award for Distinguished Research in Basic and Tumor Immunology.) Simultaneously, the American Cancer Society (ACS) announced that it was removing Coley's toxins, and two other unconventional treatments—including hyperthermia, or heat therapy—from its unproven methods list. It is hard to imagine how either immunotherapy or hyperthermia could have progressed (as both have today) while being denounced as quackery. Helen Nauts had been working towards this goal from the moment, in 1965, that the ACS had put her father's name on its black list.

In a lengthy 1991 letter to me, she pointed to the removal of Coley's toxins from the ACS list as one of her proudest achievements. She wanted me to know the details of how this came about. She confided that in 1970 she had asked Lloyd to confront the person in charge of the dreaded list, Roald N. Grant, MD, a former NYU surgeon who was then the ACS vice president in charge of "professional education." In this role, he and a science writer named Irene Bartlett had turned the ACS's monthly magazine, *CA—A Cancer Journal for Clinicians* into a scourge of medical heresy. Almost every month they exposed, debunked and virtually banned yet another unconventional treatment. The articles were then assembled into a loose-leaf book, which grew from a pamphlet to a thick volume.

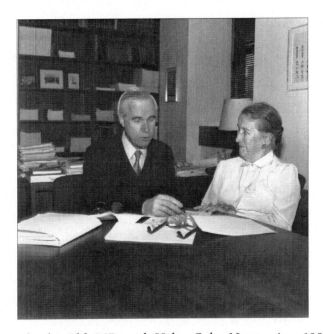

Lloyd J. Old, MD, with Helen Coley Nauts, circa 1995

In 1970, Lloyd Old phoned Grant and tried to set up a face-to-face meeting to civilly discuss the evidence for the effectiveness of Coley's toxins. But Grant was contemptuously dismissive of Coley, as he was of all 'alternative' treatments. In the same 1991 letter to me, Nauts recalled:

> *"Oh that!" [Grant] replied, in a derogatory tone, so Old decided to talk to him then and there. He did so for 45 minutes and then [Old] called me and told me about it. He said that he could feel his face getting red and his pulse rising in his anger at the man's closed mind....Five days later [Grant] died of a heart attack on the Madison Avenue bus."[35]*

Grant's sudden demise in August 1970 cleared the way for a slightly more flexible leadership. The gynecologist Sidney Arje, MD, followed as ACS's Vice President of Professional Education. Arje was no friend of unconventional methods, but was a tad more pragmatic. After five years of behind-the-scenes lobbying, ACS finally yielded. The fact that Helen had already raised one million dollars for SKI's immunology program, and that MSKCC's board chairman Laurance Rockefeller had publicly associated himself with their cause (he attended the Pierre Hotel gala) did not hurt her petition. So ACS was willing to make what seemed like a small, almost insignificant, change.

But this little change was the reason that Coley is now routinely described as the "grandfather of immunotherapy," not "that quack Coley." It made it possible for Lloyd and Helen ultimately to raise $200 million for immunology research and to "seed the field" with 1,000 investigators in tumor immunotherapy.[36] (It was also the reason that hyperthermia has been able to make slow but steady progress towards acceptance.)

The ACS never admitted to having made a mistake. And they never apologized to the many doctors whom they had undeservedly maligned or to the patients who were denied possibly useful treatments. They clung tenaciously to their position that cancer treatments could be neatly divided into two mutually exclusive categories of "proven" and "unproven." But their action spoke volumes and the Pierre Hotel gala was the watershed event.

Robert A. Good, MD, PhD

Robert Alan Good, MD, PhD, was born on May 21, 1922 in Crosby, Minnesota, the son of two teachers, Roy Herbert and Ethel Whitcomb Good. The young Bob Good decided to become a medical doctor at the age of six, after Roy died of pancreatic cancer. Ethel then raised four boys on her own in a small rented house in Minneapolis. She did an excellent job, because he and his three brothers Charles, Roy, Jr. and Thomas all received doctorates. Thomas, a pediatrician, became a professor at the University of Utah, with whom Bob Good later coauthored several scientific papers.[37]

Bob Good received his bachelor's degree and then a combined MD-PhD from the University of Minnesota, all by the age of 25. He was also triply board-certified in pediatrics, microbiology and pathology.

Among his many accomplishments, as reported in hundreds of scientific papers and book chapters, Good:

- Performed the first human bone marrow transplantation, thereby creating an entirely new branch of medicine.

- Was among the first to differentiate between human T and B lymphocytes.

- Elucidated the function of the once-neglected thymus gland.[38,39]

- Stressed the importance of the tonsils in the development of immunity, thereby reversing a 50-year trend of needlessly removing this organ.[40]

At the time I met him he was in his early 50s and was already recognized as a national leader of the "War on Cancer." There is a famous photo of him chatting with Richard Nixon at the launching of the war. Good's face was also familiar to many from the cover of *Time* magazine.

As the newly appointed president of SKI, Good initially expressed an open-minded attitude toward unconventional methods: "I'm willing to look at anything" was his mantra and laetrile was to him a scientific puzzle worthy of careful examination. One could describe his initial attitude as one of "friendly skepticism." He told *Science* that he was pleased to find that Lloyd Old and the veterinarian William D. Hardy, Jr., DVM, were already investigating laetrile in dogs when he arrived at SKI in 1972.

Such open-mindedness may strike a layperson as the unremarkable precondition for being a true scientist. But, in my opinion, it is relatively rare. Many scientists find it difficult to put aside their prejudices when it comes to scientifically investigating highly controversial areas.

Initially, Good embraced and endorsed good scientific work with laetrile. But, as president of a major scientific institution, with the whole world watching his every move, he was also by necessity and inclination a politician. He had to temper his statements, and even his thoughts, to fit the requirements of the moment. The historical record shows that when it came to laetrile, Good compromised the truth and said what was opportune, in the "pressure cooker" atmosphere that he both fostered and endured.

As I shall show, starting in January 1974 he made statements about laetrile that were simply untrue.[41] Initially, he reacted out of fear, thinking that he could remedy his misstatements with a factual report on laetrile and a clinical trial that was being contemplated in Mexico. But in fact he started a continuous chain of lies about laetrile that continues to this day. (I shall detail these lies below.)

At the same time, Good was obviously a great intellect and an enthusiastic mentor, who knew how to shower attention on talented young protégés. He encouraged "bright young minds," as he called them, and was not afraid of venturing with them into unconventional areas.

Good had the energy and accomplishments of three men, each enormously talented. He was the prolific author or co-author of 50 scientific books and 1,540 articles, still the world record. In a field filled with ambitious people, he stood out for his unparalleled drive. Some people called him the "Sammy Glick of Biology," after the heartless go-getter in Budd Schulberg's novel, *What Makes Sammy Run?*[42] But I for one never experienced this sort of pressure from him. He wanted results from his subordinates, but the goal was scientific progress, not personal aggrandizement.

Among other things, Good was a pioneer in the field of nutrition and cancer, which brought him into contact with complementary and alternative medicine (CAM). He wrote the foreword to Dr. Charles B. Simone's popular book *Cancer and Nutrition*. With two younger colleagues he explored the effects of dietary restriction on cancer incidence and survival in mice.[43]

In 1973, the MSKCC Board brought in this highly unconventional figure from the University of Minnesota to head SKI. Good was a very distinctive looking figure at the Institute. While most other scientists wore white lab coats or perhaps business suits, Good wore a turtleneck sweater, casual slacks and sneakers. (He had had polio as a child and it hurt him to walk in regular shoes.) Around his neck he wore a polished piece of silver jewelry, whose significance was a topic of lively speculation. The secretaries called it a "peace symbol" but if so, it was unlike any peace symbol I have ever seen. After he left Sloan-Kettering, I was surprised to see him wearing a standard business suit and tie, which is how you see him in most pictures on the Internet.

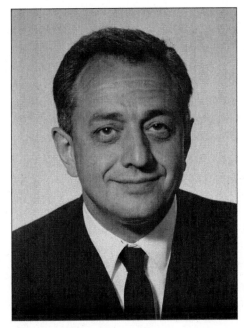

Robert A. Good, MD, PhD

It was my good fortune to begin my career as a science writer under the tutelage of this brilliant and sometimes mercurial mentor. It was from him that I first understood how a top-notch scientific mind works. That we forged a personal bond was obvious from his remark about me some years later in *Science* magazine:

> *"Moss was in a position of major trust; he knew my innermost thoughts."*[41]

Good was brimming with ideas and enthusiasm for the work being done at Sloan-Kettering and elsewhere. He himself needed to explain, convince and inspire. Something in his tone of voice told you that a cure for cancer was possible, perhaps even imminent!

He was the first to bring to my attention the work of Vilhjalmur Stefansson, the Harvard-trained anthropologist and Arctic explorer, who raised the question of whether cancer might be a "disease of civilization." He made critical but insightful remarks on this theory, as well as the work on the link between colorectal cancer and diet, which was then the pet project of the famous missionary doctor, Dennis Burkitt, MD. Burkitt had discovered the type of lymphoma that bears his name but at the time was equally famous for his theory that the Western diet was seriously deficient in fiber.[44] Good and some others invited Burkitt to speak at MSKCC in 1975, but during the talk there was open derision from some of the traditional surgeons.

When I interviewed Good, we often spoke about the exciting work on cancer immunology that he was performing along with that of Lloyd Old and their close colleague, Edward "Ted" Boyse. My boss Jerry and I jokingly dubbed them the "Good Old Boyse." I wrote so many *Center News* articles about immunology that some scientists complained that Good was monopolizing my services. But I had no hidden agenda. As I surveyed the work of SKI scientists, I found the work of Good and his collaborators to be the most interesting. Their work certainly seemed a lot more imaginative than the mind-numbing testing of tens of thousands of compounds, which was the specialty of Chester Stock.

As far as the laetrile study went, the most significant thing that Good did was to promote Lloyd Old to be his deputy director. Joseph R. Hixson,

Jr., who had preceded Jerry as Director of Public Affairs, remarked in his book, *The Patchwork Mouse*:

> *"Had Good chosen Andrew Ivy, promoter of the discredited cancer drug Krebiozen, as his deputy, the reaction of some members [of SKI] could not have been more categorically negative."*[45]

(Ivy had been the vice provost of the University of Illinois, who advocated an immune-stimulating drug, called Krebiozen, which was derived from the serum of horses inoculated with a microbe, *Actinomyces bovis.*)

Good's day began well before sunrise, and friends, colleagues and employees quickly learned to accommodate themselves to his grueling schedule. Since I lived in a two-fare zone in Sheepshead Bay, I sometimes had to get up in the wee hours to make it to one of Good's early morning meetings. And you didn't want to be late for one of these sessions! Good also thought nothing of keeping people waiting hours to see him. I took this as a sign of my lowly status until the day I saw James Watson, PhD, co-discoverer of the double helix structure of DNA, cooling his heels in Good's outer office!

The Summerlin Affair

In April 1974, the world was shocked by a major scientific scandal at Sloan-Kettering Institute. The Summerlin painted-mouse affair was a bizarre story of cheating in high places that raised serious questions about the conduct of cancer research in general and about the honesty of Sloan-Kettering's leaders in particular.

William T. Summerlin, MD, PhD (b. 1938) was a young dermatologist with a very promising future. A protégé of Dr. Good, Summerlin had been brought on board as a full member of Sloan-Kettering and also made head of a clinical department at the adjacent Memorial Hospital.[46] Most researchers spent decades working their way up the ladder, until they hopefully became full members of SKI (the Institute's equivalent of professor). So Summerlin's instant success stirred considerable resentment.

Summerlin had only half a dozen scientific papers to his credit. His éclat was due to a novel application of a technique known as tissue culturing. Starting in 1970 as a young teaching and training fellow at Stanford University, the doctor claimed to be able to take skin transplants from one individual and make them "stick" to another genetically unrelated individual.[47] He allegedly did this by culturing skin in a special medium for four to six weeks. Doing so, the samples appeared to lose their natural ability to provoke an immune response. It was just the kind of important new idea that Dr. Good loved. A medical historian has remarked, "A new era with vast promise dawned in the field of transplantation."[48]

Summerlin backed up his claims with dramatic animal work: white mice that showed dark blotches of black skin, from unrelated donor mice, on their backs. Generally, skin from one animal will not make a permanent graft to another genetically unrelated animal. After a temporary attachment it becomes inflamed, ulcerates and falls off. This is because the immune system of the receiver recognizes the new skin as foreign and rejects it. (The main exceptions to this rule are identical twins in humans and inbred strains in mice.) By "tissue culturing"—first soaking pieces of skin in a special bath—Summerlin claimed to be able to make these transplants take perfectly.

The implications of this work were revolutionary. Organ transplants can often be precarious, since the recipient's immune system may reject the new organ as foreign in short order. To prevent this, the patient is put on drugs that suppress the immune system but which, among other things, heighten one's susceptibility to cancer.

Receiving skin transplants from unrelated individuals is thus very difficult. If Summerlin's technique had been valid, skin and other organ transplants might have become relatively common and easy. Cancer patients, for example, whose disease had not spread beyond a single organ, could have received a suitable replacement—provided that replacement had first been soaked for a while in Summerlin's magic fluid. Burn victims would also have been major beneficiaries of the new technique. It was hard not to let one's mind race to the mind-boggling implications.

The Summerlin technique also had major theoretical importance. Cancer, after all, originates from normal cells but becomes a kind of foreign tissue in the body. If Summerlin had figured out what allowed the body to accept a new piece of skin as its own, perhaps others could figure out why the body of a cancer patient accepts its tumor. Clearly, then, Summerlin had a big idea.

For Summerlin himself these ideas and claims had already taken him farther than most 35-year-olds ever dream of getting: to a top post at a world-famous private research center.

Other scientists were watching Summerlin's ideas with great interest. In fact, the entire medical world was buzzing with news of the imminent breakthrough at Sloan-Kettering. *Time* magazine wrote, in a cover story on the director, "No one appreciates [its] potential more than Good..." who predicted that, as part of immunology, "it will enable us to understand the basic processes of life."[49]

Good was at Summerlin's side, directing and encouraging him, and acting as senior coauthor of his papers. Good had been brought in to firmly reestablish Sloan-Kettering as the leading cancer research center. Now he had dramatically proven his worth to Benno Schmidt and Laurance Rockefeller with this startling finding.

In the middle of 1973, however, a few scientists began to write SKI that they could not reproduce the young dermatologist's technique. Good asked Summerlin to reproduce his famous results, which he had difficulty doing—perhaps because they were faked from the start, or, less likely, because they were a one-time fluke that he didn't know how to repeat.

The showdown came on the morning of March 26, 1974. In the elevator of the Howard Building, on his way to Good's office, Summerlin quickly touched up some faded marks on a white mouse using a felt-tip pen. The touch-up job escaped Good's notice but an astute animal handler noticed the unusual patch as he was taking the mice back to their cages. Using a ball of alcohol-soaked cotton, he removed the ink markings and immediately notified several young doctors working with Summerlin.[50]

These doctors went to Good and told him of the fakery. Good in turn informed Lewis Thomas, president of the Center. The recently appointed Public Affairs director, Jerry Delaney, was also brought in on the secret. Suddenly Summerlin's spectacular breakthrough had become a major problem for the new administration. Instead of confronting the issue head-on, however, they sat on the story for weeks.

"No written word about the trouble circulated within or outside the institution," wrote Joseph Hixson in *The Patchwork Mouse*. Delaney was simply given a short statement to read to the press "in case there was a leak." As long as there was no leak, however, the administration said nothing, and there is no indication they ever intended to say anything to the public unless they were forced to do so. Finally, almost three weeks later, somebody tipped off the *New York Post* reporter, Barbara Yuncker, who broke the story in April 1974.[51]

As I was returning home by subway from a meeting at MSKCC, I glanced over the shoulder of a fellow straphanger and saw Yuncker's story on Summerlin. The headline read, "Mouse Scandal Rocks Sloan-Kettering" and I immediately thought, "Oh no, my luck! I'm signing on as the third mate on the Titanic!" But further conversations with Jerry reassured me that they would weather this storm, as they had weathered other storms in the past. At the time I knew next to nothing about their involvement with laetrile nor about the profound impact that it would have on my own life.

A peer review committee was appointed by Good himself, made up of five long-time members of the Institute: Drs. Chester Stock, Joseph Burchenal, Barney Clarkson, Martin Sonnenberg, and Edward Boyse. This committee issued a report, which gave a detailed history of the facts of the case, at least as seen from the administration's point of view. This hand-picked committee concluded that Summerlin alone was to blame for the incident. They referred to his behavior as follows:

> *"Irresponsible conduct that is incompatible with discharge of his responsibilities in the scientific community....In several instances Dr. Summerlin did indeed grossly mislead his colleagues."*[52,53]

The SKI committee attributed Summerlin's fraudulent behavior to his personal "disarray," the "desultory conduct of his everyday affairs," and other psychosocial aberrations. After lengthy consultations with lawyers, Summerlin was declared mentally unbalanced. He was dismissed but given $40,000 severance pay (one year's salary) and advised to see a psychiatrist.[54]

That July, Good and an MSKCC colleague, John L. Ninnemann, published a retraction that they hoped would put the whole scientific controversy to rest.[55] Summerlin went off to practice as a dermatologist in Bentonville, Arkansas and never faced any charges from the medical society or the state. By all accounts, he has had an unremarkable career for the past 35 years. The peer review committee blamed Good for prematurely promoting Summerlin, but exonerated him of any direct responsibility for the deception, although he was senior author on Summerlin's papers.[56,57,58]

Science magazine reporter Barbara J. Culliton summarized the sense of dismay in the scientific community:

> *"There is no sin in science more grievous than falsifying data. There is no accusation that can be made against a man more serious than that he is guilty of such a sin. The very thought of fakery threatens the powerful mystique of the purity of science. It stirs deep and contradictory feelings of incredulity, outrage, and remorse among the entire scientific community—feelings it is experiencing now in the very complex and unresolved matter of William T. Summerlin."*[59]

Prominent scientists at the time noted that "the episode reflected dangerous trends in current efforts to gain scientific acclaim and funds for research, as well as the possible misdirection of research at Sloan-Kettering itself."[60]

Where in all this was the SKI Board of Scientific Consultants, a gathering of experts who were supposed to oversee and thereby prevent malfeasance at this prestigious institution? The Nobel Prize winner Sir Peter Medawar (1915-1987) was chairman of the SKI Board of Scientific

Consultants at the time. He later explained why, despite his strong doubts, he did not say anything to contradict Summerlin's claims:

> *"I simply lacked the moral courage to say at the time that I thought we were the victims of a hoax or a confidence trick. It is easy in theory to say these things, but in practice very senior scientists do not like trampling on their juniors in public."*[61]

The whole business was revealing of the way frauds and cover-ups could be perpetrated in high places. *Science* concluded :

> *"Sloan-Kettering, these days, is not a happy place. It is rich and getting richer, but not happy.... It appears that a high-pressure environment that drives individuals to exaggeration and fosters hostility is not ideal for the kind of achievements in research that Good, like everyone else, would like to see."*[62]

Summerlin himself later charged that there was a "pressure-cooker atmosphere" at SKI. He blamed his problems on the "frenetic situation" at the Institute and especially on the "extreme pressure put on me by the Institute director [Good, ed.] to publicize information...."[63]

The Summerlin affair was a major embarrassment for Sloan-Kettering, and especially for its new director. It put a damper on enthusiasm for radically new directions of research and reestablished the position of the conservative members who had viewed Good's ascendancy to the directorship of "their" institution with trepidation.[64]

My first assignment at MSKCC was to carry out some "private eye" digging into Summerlin's personal history. Jerry told me that the administration wanted to dig up some 'dirt' on him that they might use as leverage should he decide to implicate them in his misdeeds. So I spent a few days making phone calls to Summerlin's former employers and colleagues, but I could find nothing in his past that was noteworthy. I do remember sitting there that first day, wondering if this job was really for me. Skullduggery seemed at odds with the rewarding intellectual work that I had signed on to do.

Sloan-Kettering was also approaching a financial crisis, caused in part by the new administration's extravagant spending on expensive projects. A discovery of this magnitude would have attracted abundant cash and would have rescued the institution. Rockefeller and Schmidt wanted a Nobel laureate to head their institution (they later got one in Harold Varmus, MD) and Good had every reason to expect a Nobel Prize. Summerlin's work would have put him over the top.

Lewis Thomas, MD

Lewis Thomas, MD, was born on November 25, 1913, in Flushing, NY, the son of a family physician and his nurse wife. Before coming to MSKCC he had been dean of the medical schools at Yale University and NYU. Thomas was the president of SKI's parent corporation, Memorial Sloan-Kettering Cancer Center and was therefore the top spokesperson for MSKCC.

Thomas had an engaging literary personality and a unique style of making esoteric topics come alive to those on the humanities side of the "Two Cultures."[65] He had a felicitous way of turning a phrase. His writing especially evoked the smallness of man in the cosmos. He wrote that "the mere fact of our existence should keep us all in a state of contented dazzlement" and that "the greatest of all the accomplishments of 20th century science has been the discovery of human ignorance."[66]

How could one not be drawn to a great man who was aware of his own ignorance and insignificance? I looked forward to our interactions. But the Lewis Thomas I experienced was quite different from his literary persona. He gave as little as humanly possible to those in a subordinate position and visiting him was almost physically painful.

When we in Public Affairs moved out of our 62nd St. offices and into the new hospital, I hoped it might lead to a closer relationship with Thomas. Our office was just one floor below his offices on the 21st floor, but what a distance that represented. One problem was that Jerry Delaney guarded his personal and professional relationship with Thomas. On the few occasions that Jerry took me along to interview Thomas, the great man remained Sphinx-like, answering questions with terse monosyllables. His gaze, through thick glasses, seemed bored or disdainful.

I once got onto the elevator immediately after him and heartily wished him a good morning…but he just stared straight through me. This happened on a second occasion as well. I felt hurt and I also worried that perhaps I had somehow offended him. Then one day I heard two secretaries whisper, as Thomas exited the elevator, "He's so stuck up. He never says hello to anyone." I then felt much better, as I saw it was nothing personal. He was not friendly to underlings, unless perhaps he had a particular use for them.

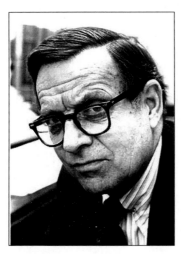

Lewis Thomas, MD

In 1972, he assured Benno Schmidt, "This institution can answer the laetrile question fairly quickly." Perhaps he let his true feelings show in October 1973 with this snide remark to *Science*:

> "*These are bad times for Reason, all around. Suddenly, all of the major ills are being coped with by acupuncture. If not acupuncture, it is apricot pits.*"[67]

Laetrile was of course derived from apricot "pits" or, rather, kernels. This wasn't a good omen.

But on the surface, at least, the new leaders of MSKCC had agreed to test laetrile without prejudice. They had the resources. They had the brains.

The main question was whether they had the courage to stick by their conclusions, wherever these led.

Three Experimentalists

ood, Thomas and Old were the public mouthpieces of the institution, but they did not actually do any laetrile experiments. The
controversy over laetrile at SKI revolved around the activities of
half a dozen people, but particularly three key men: Kanematsu Sugiura,
DSc; his immediate supervisor, SKI vice president C. Chester Stock, PhD;
and his main antagonist, Catholic Medical Center's Daniel S. Martin, MD.
It is therefore essential that the reader obtain a full picture of these three,
and especially of the man who did most of the experiments discussed in
this book. If "a man's character is his fate," as the Greek philosopher Hera-
clitus said, then many features of this story derive from their character,
and especially from the moral courage of one man.

Kanematsu Sugiura, DSc

I first met Kanematsu Sugiura in the summer of 1974. New to the job, I
was looking for promising topics to write about for our monthly publication, *Center News*. (It still exists as a bimonthly online magazine.) My
boss, Jerry Delaney, suggested that I go to the Walker Laboratory in Rye,
NY, to troll for story ideas.

The Walker Lab had opened in 1959 on the grounds of a large estate on
the Boston Post Road. Its construction was part of a $12 million gift from
the stockbroker Donald Stone Walker, and was dedicated to the study of
chemotherapy in test tubes, fertilized eggs and animals. At the time of its
dedication the director of NCI's chemotherapy service described the
Walker facility as "the finest in the world."[68]

But by 1974, Walker employees felt neglected by their "downtown" SKI
counterparts. The sudden ascendancy of the immunology program put the
systematic search for chemical treatments (their specialty) in doubt. Walker
scientists felt insecure and under-appreciated. Because of their geographic
isolation, their work was inadequately recognized in *Center News*. As it
turned out, they had good reason to be concerned, because a few years later
SKI sold off the facility for its 44 acres of precious Westchester real estate.

A station wagon left the Kettering Laboratory on East 68th Street every workday morning for the half hour trip to Rye; it returned every afternoon at 3 pm. One fine summer day in 1974 I rode up to Rye with Chester Stock, head of the Walker facility, who had arranged for us to have lunch with some of the leading figures there. Among these was an elderly Japanese-American scientist, Kanematsu Sugiura, who sat upright throughout, dressed rather formally in a white lab coat over shirt and tie. He had a pleasant but almost mask-like demeanor and seemed polite, modest and self-contained.

Although he wrote English elegantly—as evidenced by hundreds of scientific papers—he spoke with a Japanese accent, and I sometimes had to strain to understand him. Like many older people, he was also slightly hard of hearing. Stock and others at the Walker Lab seemed to have a genuine affection for their older colleague.

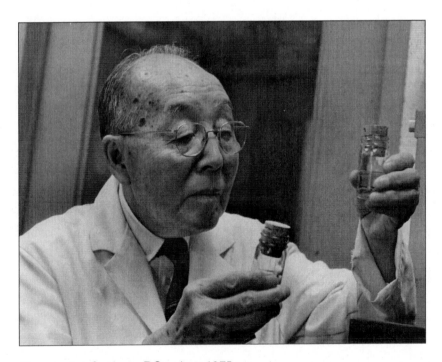

Kanematsu Sugiura, DSc, circa 1975

Stock and Sugiura shared something else. They had appeared together (along with the late SKI Director Cornelius P. "Dusty" Rhoads) on the June

1973 cover of *Cancer Research*. This was a keystone achievement, arguably more prestigious for a scientist than being on the cover of *Time* magazine (as three past MSKCC directors, Ewing, Rhoads, and Good, had been).

On the shuttle back to New York City, Stock agreed (although I sensed some hesitation) that a biographical portrait of Sugiura for *Center News* would be a good idea. I therefore made an appointment to return in a few weeks to interview Sugiura again.

On this return visit I found him in the second floor office that he shared with the scientist Isabel Morgan Mountain, PhD, daughter of the Nobel laureate T. H. Morgan.[69] Sugiura had officially retired in 1962 at age 70, yet he continued to work steadily. Every day, Monday to Friday, and when required on Saturdays and Sunday as well, Sugiura arrived at the three-story suburban building at 8:00 am. Every day at precisely 5:00 pm he left for his home in nearby Harrison, NY in the company of his son-in-law and fellow SKI employee, Franz Schmid, DVM (who was married to Sugiura's daughter, Miyono).

As an example of his legendary patience, one of the laetrile experiments we are about to discuss required him to inject and observe mice every day, seven days a week. Sugiura kept up this regimen, never missing a single day or wavering in his duty, for two-and-a-half years!

To me, Sugiura embodied the best of the Japanese character. He was like one of those Japanese persons deemed a "Living National Treasure." These are outstanding individuals, mainly in the crafts or performing arts, who have attained an unusually high degree of mastery in their chosen field. Sugiura was that type of individual, although his medium was of course not paper folding, but laboratory science, specifically the experimental chemotherapy of cancer.[70]

Sugiura was born in the small town of Tsushima (west of Nagoya, in Aichi Prefecture) on June 5, 1892. In 1906, after Japan won the Russo-Japanese War, the American railroad tycoon E.H. Harriman arrived to purchase the captured trans-Manchurian railway. Kanematsu's older brother, Kamasaburo, was appointed the official interpreter and guide for Mr. Harriman.[71]

The railroad transaction fell through, but Harriman was intrigued by an exhibition that Kamasaburo had arranged of the traditional arts of ken-jitsu (swordsmanship) and jiu-jitsu (martial arts). Considering the performers a novel form of amusement, Harriman decided to bring half a dozen of them from the Kodokan Judo Institute of Kyoto to the US for a six-month visit.

Jiu-jitsu was of course more than an "entertainment novelty," as Harriman called it. There were and are profound philosophical principles at its root, such as "defeating strength through flexibility" and "maximum efficient use of physical and mental energy." These qualities were to serve Sugiura well in the course of his long life, including in his late-in-life struggles.

In October 1905, a team of six jiu-jitsu performers sailed with the Harriman family aboard the luxurious *Siberia Maru*, bound for San Francisco. These were the first Japanese martial artists to reach North American shores and among them was a 13-year-old prodigy named Kanematsu Sugiura.

The other performers lodged at a Japanese inn in New York City, but Sugiura, being underage, lived with Harriman's personal physician, William G. Lyle, MD. In 1906 these judokas (judo practitioners) performed at the White House for Teddy Roosevelt, who was America's first brown belt, as well to enthusiastic crowds at Columbia University and elsewhere.[72]

The *New York Times* described this team as "E.H. Harriman's troupe of six clever wrestlers and swordsmen."[73] The paper commented:

> *"Mr. Harriman during his late visit to Japan was so much interested in the art of jiu-jitsu as practiced by the most experienced members of that science that he brought to America a troupe of six of the most skillful Japanese performers...They are all skillful acrobats, and the rapidity with which they handle the short swords makes the customary fencing seen by our amateur foilsmen appear very tame."[74]*

The *Times* described Kanematsu as "a lad of about 13 years of age." Although by far the smallest, he amazed American audiences by his ability to "tumble a man twice his size and strength in a matter of seconds without bodily injury to either."[75]

Harriman's plan was to educate all of the Japanese performers, American-style. The *New York Times* reported:

> *"Besides giving exhibitions of their skill, the Japs [sic!] are going to be educated here, and in the near future will probably enter one of our colleges, as soon as their command of the English language becomes sufficiently perfect to read the college text books and understand the lectures."*[76]

But after six months, the entire team was afflicted by homesickness and went home, except Kanematsu, who stayed on as the houseguest of Lyle. On my first visit to him in 1974, he proudly showed me pictures of himself as a handsome, athletic young man, standing barefoot in the snow in his kendo (Japanese fencing) uniform.[77]

Although Kanematsu also was homesick, he knew this was the only way he would be able to get an education. The youngest of seven children, he was left fatherless when the elder Sugiura, a dye maker, had succumbed to stomach cancer.[78] Although a bright student, his family could not afford to continue his schooling and had apprenticed him to a hardware business. Harriman's largesse offered him a better future.

In New York City, Sugiura attended Public School No. 69 and Townsend Harris High School. The latter was a legendary incubator of talented youngsters whose parents could not afford to send them to elite private schools. Its alumni were to include famous scientists (Jonas Salk), jurists (Felix Frankfurter), entertainers (Richard Rogers) and politicians (Adam Clayton Powell).

Sugiura's interest in science began early. After school hours, he worked at Roosevelt Hospital, where he washed instruments, scrubbed containers, and generally helped doctors with their experiments.

In 1909 Harriman himself died of stomach cancer and left $1 million to establish a cancer research laboratory at Roosevelt Hospital. Lyle, who had attended Harriman on his deathbed, became its first director, and that is how, in 1911, young Kanematsu was hired as assistant chemist at the Harriman Research Laboratory.

In 1912, he began his first experiments in the chemotherapy of cancer under Richard Weil, MD, chairman of Experimental Medicine at Cornell University Medical College. With scholarship funds provided by the Harriman family, Kanematsu attended evening classes at the Polytechnic Institute of Brooklyn, receiving his Bachelor of Science degree in chemistry there in 1915. Through summer classes at Columbia University he then completed the requirements for a Master of Arts degree in Chemistry in 1917.[79] By this time, he had already authored 14 scientific papers.

In the pre-World War I days, when there were no animal supply houses, Sugiura would find animals with spontaneous tumors by scouring pet stores in New York City. He told me that he would also catch rats by hunting in the basement of Roosevelt Hospital. He began by testing various inorganic compounds on cancerous animals and was able to demonstrate that such chemicals had a small, but real, anticancer effect. Such findings helped overcome widespread skepticism about chemotherapy and spurred interest in finding yet more active chemicals.

In 1917, the Harriman family lost interest in cancer and turned its attention to politics. The Harriman Research Laboratory closed its doors, and staff members were told to seek positions elsewhere. E. H. Harriman's son, William Averell Harriman, later became Democratic governor of New York.

In November 1917, Memorial Hospital's director, James Ewing, MD (1866-1943), decided to expand the hospital's tumor transplantation program, and hired Sugiura. This was an unprecedented opportunity for Sugiura to study cancer under the microscope. Although surgical pathology had its roots in 19th century Germany, it has a long and distinguished history in the US as well. "The Chief," as Ewing was called, was the first professor of Pathology at Cornell University, one of the founders of the American Association for Cancer Research (AACR), and gave his name to Ewing's sarcoma, a type of bone cancer.[80]

Sugiura progressed to studies of radiation, nutrition, enzyme therapy, tumor transplantation, experimental chemotherapy, and carcinogenesis. A close colleague, Dorris Hutchison, PhD, later wrote:

> "*His test results in experimental chemotherapy encompass every type of chemical and biological agent received at the Sloan-Kettering Institute.... Sugiura did as Ewing asked and more. He became a 'jack of all trades,' biochemist, radiologist, pharmacist, photographer, and 'evening' pathologist at Dr. Ewing's side.*"[81]

Later, Sugiura worked closely with Cornelius P. "Dusty" Rhoads, MD, who would become first president of Sloan-Kettering Institute. Prior to laetrile, his one brush with fame had been experiments showing that a synthetic dye known as "butter yellow" could cause cancer[82] but that the B vitamin riboflavin could partially prevent cancer formation.[83,84] But throughout his long life Sugiura proved himself disinterested in publicity. He was a laboratory scientist par excellence, content if he were left alone to do his work.

Then came World War II. Despite the fact that he had lived productively in his adopted country for decades, and had a daughter born in the US, Sugiura, as a Japanese living in a US coastal area, was threatened with internment in a camp. Intervention by Rhoads at the "highest levels of government"[85] prevented this and Sugiura was "only" placed under house arrest.[86] Nothing could keep him from his work, however, and, at great risk to himself, he would "wander away" from his apartment on the Grand Concourse in the Bronx in order to do research at the old Memorial Hospital on Central Park West and West 105th St.

After the war, the research structure at Memorial Hospital changed. Whereas previously the scientific as well as the clinical work had been done at Memorial Hospital, laboratory research was transferred to the newly formed Sloan-Kettering Institute (SKI). In 1953, he became a naturalized American citizen. Sugiura was made an associate member of SKI in 1947 and a full member (equivalent to a full professor) in 1959.

Sugiura's official title was head of the Solid Tumor Section of Sloan-Kettering's Division of Experimental Chemotherapy. He also served as the Institute's official liaison with Japanese scientists, including those visiting the US. Japan was then an important source of new anticancer drugs, and he worked on a new antibiotic/anticancer agent from Japan, mitomycin C.[87]

Over the course of his long life Sugiura received many honors. In 1925, the Kyoto Imperial University awarded him an honorary Doctorate of Science (DSc) degree. In that same year he received the Leonard Prize of the Roentgen Society for his work on radiation biology. In 1960 the Japanese government honored him for his cultural services and in the same year Emperor Hirohito awarded him membership in the Order of the Sacred Treasure, Third Class. In 1965, the Japan Medical Association presented him with its highest award for outstanding contributions to cancer research and "for his services, an inspiration to so many Japanese physicians and surgeons." In 1966, New York City Mayor John V. Lindsay and the New York County Medical Society recognized him for his cultural services and his dedication to the field of medicine.

The first of his 250 PubMed-indexed papers and book chapters appeared in 1922 (other non-PubMed papers had appeared earlier).[88] His last paper was published in the Japanese cancer journal, *Gann*, in 1978. His work thus spanned 60 years of chemotherapy research and touched on all the chief areas of progress. He was particularly interested, said his long-time colleague Dorris Hutchison, PhD, in "the development of new animal tumor models," the very topic that would come to the fore in the laetrile debate.

He was also a consummate teacher of young experimentalists. It was in recognition of this activity that a photograph of him teaching graduate students was featured on the cover of Bristol-Myers Squibb's *A Century of Oncology, A Photographic History of Cancer Research*.[89]

In 1962 he formally retired and became Member Emeritus. Three years later, Stock helped gather Sugiura's papers into a four-volume *Collected Works*. In words that would come back to haunt him, Stock summarized the scientific world's opinion:

"Few, if any, names in cancer research are as widely known as Kanematsu Sugiura's…. Possibly the high regard in which his work is held, is best characterized by a comment made to me by a visiting investigator in cancer research from Russia. He said, 'When Dr. Sugiura publishes, we know we don't have to repeat the study, for we would obtain the same results he has reported'."[90]

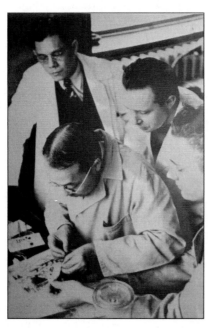

Sugiura teaching mouse examination techniques, circa 1950

Sugiura had lived a long and full life, been honored by his peers, and was respected in both his adopted and native land. By every indication, he would end his life as peacefully as he had lived it, content with his half-page niche in *Contrary to Nature,* the official National Cancer Institute-sponsored history of cancer research.[91]

Yet at age 80, Sugiura found himself in the center of a furious controversy. Because he had done what he was told, and recorded what he saw, he lived to see old friends desert him, a close relative fail to support him, and former colleagues question his sanity and competence.

What Sugiura did was agree, in the summer of 1972, to test laetrile in spontaneously occurring tumors in mice.

In assessing Sugiura's role in the laetrile controversy one must answer the question of whether a person who had faithfully served his profession, institution and adopted country for 60 years, who had retired honorably with a good pension, and whose entire social circle consisted of members of that Institute, would suddenly seek to embarrass all his friends, relatives and colleagues by radically misrepresenting his own findings?

This was of course absurd. He would have to have been flaky, inconsistent or erratic and he was the opposite of those things, the very picture of a careful and scrupulous scientist. Even his harshest critics ascribed his positive results with laetrile to some vaguely conceived "unconscious bias" rather than any conscious inclination towards malice aforethought. As we seek for any possible source of pro-laetrile bias, we should remember that it was SKI officials (particularly Old and Stock) who asked him to conduct the laetrile experiments in question...he did not volunteer, having shown no prior interest in the topic. Sugiura undertook this job with the same craftsman-like diligence that he undertook any task to which he was assigned. And had the topic not been laetrile it is doubtful that his findings would have generated the slightest controversy.

As the controversy progressed, however, Sloan-Kettering's leaders repeatedly underestimated Sugiura's tenacious belief in the inviolability of scientific findings.

"Throughout his life, Dr. Sugiura held fast to his convictions," said Dorris Hutchison, with a nod toward the laetrile controversy. By upholding the accuracy of his meticulous observations, in the face of furious opposition, Sugiura alienated many people, including his main supporters at SKI. But he held true to his fundamental principle, which he summarized in five brief words: "I write what I see."

A person in Sugiura's position typically shows a powerful "bias" towards the urgent demands of his employers, family and friends. One thinks of Upton Sinclair's dictum, "It is impossible to get a man to understand something if his livelihood depends on him not understanding."[92] In other words, we typically do not bite the hand that feeds us. This would have been compounded by his national origin. A British ambassador to Japan once said that in Japanese society "loyalty is the supreme virtue." He continued:

> *"Loyalty to Japan and to the emperor was inculcated into every child in prewar Japan. The emphasis now seems to be on loyalty to the company employing you, loyalty to your section in the company and loyalty to your immediate colleagues."*[93]

Therefore, everything in Sugiura's background cried out for him to obey the wishes of his "superiors." This would have been reinforced by his training in jiu-jitsu. Its principles include bowing to one's teachers, never questioning the instructor's decisions, respecting and obeying all orders, and always answering your teacher with a crisp, "Yes, sensei!"[94]

The fact that Sugiura defied authority in this case speaks volumes about the strength with which he held to his belief in his own findings concerning laetrile. Any personal consideration was overridden by his steadfast commitment to the truth. I repeatedly saw proof of this dedication. He would not tell even a white lie in order to save a friend from embarrassment. I took to calling him "compulsively" or even "pathologically honest," because of this unbending dedication to the truth.

C. Chester Stock, PhD

Before discussing the outcome of Sugiura's laetrile experiments, it is necessary to introduce another important figure in the laetrile saga, and that was Sugiura's friend-turned-antagonist, SKI's vice president C. Chester Stock, PhD.

Charles Chester Stock was born in Terre Haute, Indiana, on May 10, 1910. He was a graduate of Garfield High School and received a chemical engineering degree from Rose Polytechnic Institute (now the Rose-Hulman Institute of Technology), where his father, Orion L. Stock, taught drawing.[95]

In 1937 Stock received a doctorate in physiological chemistry from Johns Hopkins University, Baltimore, and in 1941 a master's degree in medical bacteriology from New York University. In 1947, he became chief of chemotherapy research at the newly organized Sloan-Kettering Institute and in 1961 became its first named vice president. In 1965, he received the Alfred P. Sloan award for cancer research.

For most of his career, Stock was a steady and reliable administrator, who accumulated numerous publications, awards and honors, but never to my knowledge did anything memorable in science.

At the time I met him, he headed the Division of Experimental Chemotherapy at Sloan-Kettering and also ran the Walker Laboratory. Despite the lack of conspicuous success in finding new cancer drugs, Stock on the whole was respected as an efficient and workman-like supervisor of a massive research project. When he retired in 1980, Sloan-Kettering named the annual C. Chester Stock Award Lectureship after him.

Technically speaking, Sugiura worked under him, although he was senior both in terms of age and experience. In fact, Stock was basically an administrator who relied on his staff to do the actual work. Stock owed much of his success at SKI to Sugiura.

From my experience, Stock was not a man who showed much emotion, other than occasional flashes of anger and annoyance. For instance, in the three-plus years that I knew him I saw him grimace a few times but never saw him smile.

Although his job eventually included finding ways to undermine Sugiura's credibility, he seemed pained to do so. I believe his personal affection for Sugiura was genuine (as paradoxical as that might seem).

In the ordinary course of events, Stock was a factual man. Yet in the course of the laetrile struggle, he became mired deeper and deeper in a cover-up that, initially at least, was not of his making. Eventually, as I shall show, he lied outright about the outcome of the testing. Equally ludicrous was how he endorsed an eccentric procedure (Martin's bioassay) that at other times he would have greeted with the utmost skepticism. (Martin's bioassay will be described in full detail below.) But by 1975 he had a deeply distasteful job to do and proceeded in his methodical way, despite any personal qualms he harbored about doing so.

Stock was, in essence, a company man. His overwhelming priority was his loyalty to Sloan-Kettering, the institute that had provided him with both his sense of purpose and his high social status. In mid-1975, he got on board the anti-laetrile bandwagon and then did everything in his power to keep this issue from harming his beloved institution.

Daniel S. Martin, MD

At the time that Daniel S. Martin, MD became influential in the laetrile studies at Sloan-Kettering he was not even a member of the staff. He was a surgeon and owner of a mouse-breeding business in Woodhaven, Queens.

As early as 1968, writing in *CA,* the ACS journal that introduced the *Unproven Methods* series, Martin exposed an extreme animus towards what is now called complementary and alternative medicine (CAM). He warned clinicians (the main audience for that journal) as a matter of policy not to always tell patients the truth about their cancer. He counseled:

> *"The truth should be told, but not necessarily the whole truth...."*[96]

For example, he said, patients should not be told that their cancer might recur. They should be counseled "without reference to the possibility of unknown spread of the disease."[97] He was also among those zealots who recommended the use of highly toxic chemotherapy, even when it was known to be ineffective, as a way of keeping patients away from "all sorts of new treatments" and "quacks who take the patient's last savings to no avail."[98]

The image of a cancer patient being given chemotherapy of known ineffectiveness in order to achieve not a medical but a social end (keeping him away from quackery) is not a pleasant one.

Martin emerged as a kind of "anti-Sugiura" in the SKI laetrile saga. Animated by a bitter hatred of "quackery," Martin constructed an elaborate framework to explain why Sugiura was wrong, he was right, and laetrile not only did not work but *could* not work.

In the mid-1970s Martin became an outspoken opponent of what he called the "laetrile hoax."[99] He would issue quotable 'sound bites' at meetings, debates and in *New York Times* op-eds. In 1976, he even went to the trouble of mimeographing an anti-laetrile tract. Some of his choice quotations were as follows:

- "I flatfootedly and categorically tell you that laetrile is without activity against spontaneous tumors in mice—period." —*Medical World News*, 1975.[100]

- Laetrile is "a swindle, a hoax, a fraud and a rip-off. The only thing it can do is take your money." —Speaking at the FDA's Kansas City hearings on laetrile, May 1977.[101]

- "Laetrile has been found absolutely devoid of activity, period. It's just that simple." —Speaking at the SKI Press Conference, June 1977.

Martin's initial involvement with laetrile came about because he had a ready supply of mice that spontaneously developed tumors of the breast. He had created this so-called CD8F1 mouse by crossing two other mouse strains that spontaneously developed breast cancer. Martin created this model because he believed in the superiority of spontaneous over transplantable tumors, which is why Lloyd Old initially saw him as a potential ally. An added plus was that Martin's colony was located across the East River in nearby Queens, at a time when there were not many sources of such mice.

But Martin had his own agenda. By being the sole source of these mice, he could work his way into SKI's laetrile testing program. He made no secret of the fact that he wanted to obtain a staff position at MSKCC. A long-term goal was to get the CD8F1 mouse adopted as a standard screening tool for new drugs at NCI.[102]

Martin's transformation from mouse supplier to key player took place in 1975. As late as 1974 the NCI had disdainfully turned down his grant application and dismissed the importance of his mouse colony as "obscure."

> "I sincerely hope that you will find a mechanism to accomplish your goal," Dr. Dorothy B. Windhorst, MD, speaking for the NCI, frostily told him.[103]

He was conspicuously absent from a key meeting on laetrile held at the FDA in July 1974 (see below). But shortly thereafter, after his opposition to laetrile became clear, NCI reconsidered, and in the spring of 1975, its officials abruptly reversed their decision and gave Martin $1 million to support a colony of 3,000 CD8F1 mice. The goal (according to *Medical World News*) was to allow the laetrile studies to go forward.[104]

So, at the height of the laetrile struggle, Martin received the equivalent of $4.3 million in today's dollars to breed what Dorothy Windhorst had months earlier called his "obscure" mice.[105] This grant coincided with the start of his vitriolic campaign against laetrile.

Although Martin's influence over SKI's laetrile studies was baleful, he was a contradictory figure, who also had some progressive features.

Dr. Martin was born Daniel Martin Shapiro in Brooklyn, New York on October 29, 1921. His father, Jacob, was a dentist, and his mother, Rose, a homemaker. In his first paper, from 1949, he listed himself as a captain in the Marine Corps.[106]

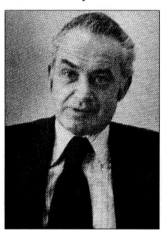

Daniel S. Martin, MD, circa 1977

He published 20 scientific papers under his birth name when, for reasons unknown, at age 37, he changed his name to "Daniel S. Martin." His peripatetic career led him from Columbia University's College of Physicians and Surgeons,[107] to New England Deaconess Hospital in Boston, to Florida's Jackson Memorial Hospital, to the University of Miami, and then back to New York's Catholic Medical Center, and finally to Memorial

Sloan-Kettering.[108,109,110] With the merger, bankruptcy and finally the total liquidation of the Catholic Medical Center came the sale of Martin's cherished CD8F1 mouse colony to a firm in Alabama.[111] In 1986 this mouse colony was liquidated and it passed into history. Martin himself died in an automobile accident near his home in Pound Ridge, NY, on July 5, 2005.

On the positive side, Martin was an early proponent of using adjuvant chemotherapy after surgery,[112] and wrote a book chapter on that topic as early as 1969.[113] This was considered quite unusual at the time. He was also an early advocate of immunotherapy, when that discipline had few friends in oncology.[114]

Even today, his work of the 1950s is sometimes cited, along that of other pioneers, as instrumental in overturning the outdated theories of Prof. William S. Halsted:

> *"Halsted's notion would have remained unquestioned were it*
> *not for the work of Daniel Martin Shapiro...and colleagues*
> *who built a compelling alternative theory from the*
> *observation that patients without axillary lymph-node*
> *involvement could still develop distant metastases."*[115]

In the late 1960s Martin and his long-time coworker, Ruth Adele Fugmann, PhD, moved from Florida back to New York City.[116] There, Martin became Chairman of the Department of Surgery at the Catholic Medical Center (CAMC) of Brooklyn and Queens. On paper, Martin had attained a department chairmanship in the Big Apple with space to house his colony of CD8F1 mice. In reality, however, the CAMC was near the bottom of the pecking order in New York medicine.

The CAMC administration soon ran up against Martin's abrasive personality. Not long after his arrival, furious clashes began, and finally the governing Joint Conference Committee fired him as chairman of the surgery department. (They were contractually obligated to retain him as a surgeon.) He sued for breach of contract and, in the turmoil surrounding his lawsuit, his scientific work all but ground to a halt. Generally a prolific author, between 1971 and 1974, he appeared as coauthor of just a single scientific paper.[117]

I n 1973, the New York Supreme Court upheld the legality of Martin's firing.[118] Associate Justice Francis T. Murphy took note of the "open animosity displayed by a majority of the members of the Joint Conference Committee" towards Martin. In December 1974, the Court of Appeals upheld the lower court's decision. It also pointed to broader problems:

> *"It is evident that [Martin] and his department had been*
> *embroiled for some time in contention with other*
> *departments in the Medical Center...he had been in running*
> *conflict with the lay director of medical affairs and the lay*
> *board of trustees."[119]*

Martin, the Appeals Court admonished, "misconstrues the function of the Joint Conference Committee, his appearance before it, and the manner in which it was composed." The Appeals Court revealed that Martin had been "removed to a building long discontinued as a hospital and used only for limited administrative and research purposes." This building was St. Anthony's, a Victorian era tuberculosis hospital that had been shuttered since 1966. But a section of this graffiti-covered, "unkempt eyesore,"[120] as it was called locally, was reopened to house Martin and his mouse colony. The Appeals Court vividly described this abandoned facility as "a Siberia."[121]

After that, the survival of the CD8F1 mouse facility was perpetually in doubt. Martin, abhorred by the leaders of his own institution, and "embroiled in contention" with other department heads, as the judge put it, had failed to interest the NCI in funding an expansion of his "obscure" facility.[122]

He had zero success in selling his rodent model to anyone else in the scientific community. Then, suddenly, in mid-1972, his fortunes abruptly changed. He received a call from Sloan-Kettering Institute—that wealthy institution towering over the East River—asking him to supply mice for its laetrile experiments. Martin saw a chance to repair his failing career. Sloan-Kettering was not only a potential customer for his mice, but, more importantly, their use of CD8F1 mice in this high profile study raised the possibility that NCI would adopt it more broadly. This could lead to enormous sales worldwide.

In addition, if he could sell the scientific world on the concept of using a companion test called a "bioassay," that would automatically double or triple his sales. That was because only female mice were used in breast tumor experiments, while male mice had to be sacrificed. But since the bioassay involved transplanting tumors from each female into two additional male mice he had discovered a use for these otherwise wasted rodents.

Another uptick in his fortunes occurred when Martin, embracing the mantle of a 'quackbuster,' became chairman of the Subcommittee on Unorthodox Therapies of the American Society of Clinical Oncology (ASCO). Quackbusters are inveterate opponents of complementary and alternative medicine whose name was ultimately derived from a cartoon, *Daffy Duck's Quackbusters*. This immediately brought him to national prominence as the leader of other vehement opponents of laetrile, such as Irving J. Lerner, MD and Jerry P. Lewis, MD of the University of California, Davis. Together, these subcommittee members wrote a pamphlet, *Ineffective Cancer Therapies: A Guide for the Layperson*.[123]

This tract presupposed the ineffectiveness of laetrile and other treatments discussed within it. It was as uniformly negative as anything that came from the pen of the original quackbuster, Dr. Victor Herbert of the Bronx Veterans Administration (VA) hospital. This was no coincidence, since Herbert was the Subcommittee's chief consultant. In their discussion of laetrile, Martin and the others employed the characteristic slash-and-burn style of Dr. Herbert. But the Subcommittee did not include a single person sympathetic towards any of the non-conventional approaches under discussion.

Martin took to his role as a quackbuster with great gusto, with a steady stream of television appearances, magazine articles, newspaper interviews, letters to editors, and op-eds in the *New York Times* and elsewhere. His writing style was cliché-ridden but serviceable enough for the anti-laetrile crusade.

For example, in a June 11, 1977 article, which appeared the weekend before the SKI press conference, Martin vented his spleen against laetrile, calling it in rapid succession a "quack cancer nostrum...worthless... unproved...dangerous deception... illusion..." and so forth.[124] In an interview with a syndicated columnist Ben Zinser, Martin called laetrile a "cunning, money-making fraud."[125] Like Herbert, he appeared in court as an "expert witness" against laetrile-using doctors, such as Congressman Larry Macdonald, MD (D-GA).[126]

Martin reduced this complex issue to a contest between "quackery" and "science," which was a variant on his black-vs.-white, good-vs.-evil, us-vs.-them way of thinking.[127] *Science's* Nicholas Wade, after interviewing him in November 1977, called him a "zealous and vocal antagonist of laetrile."[128]

Martin had no compunctions about falsely declaring that all studies of laetrile had been negative, and would always necessarily be so.[129] Even if we grant that Martin ardently believed his own studies to have been negative, it was almost unprecedented for a scientist to utterly negate the work of more experienced colleagues, such as SKI's Dr. Sugiura.

At the June 1977 SKI press conference, Martin engaged in a passive-aggressive rant over the media's refusal to acknowledge that laetrile had allegedly failed a clinical trial in Mexico and had consequently been banned there. Buttonholing a TV cameraman, Martin began a rambling disputation:

> *"The Mexican government has announced that their own physicians, after evaluating laetrile clinically... have stated that laetrile lacked efficacy as an anticancer agent. That's an official statement by the Mexican government. It's been released to the press repeatedly by myself, by the FDA, by the State Department of the United States, and yet there hasn't been one single follow through by the media....*
>
> *"You've got a definitive clinical trial in the country that's been sending laetrile to us across the border repeatedly and now says it's no good."[130]*

The part about a Mexican "clinical trial" was untrue. There is no record of any clinical trial with laetrile ever taking place in Mexico. But laetrile has been in continuous use there since 1963, and in fact is still employed as part of the treatment regimen in half a dozen clinics in the Tijuana area. What Martin apparently was referring to was a letter that the US State Department solicited from the Mexican government, stating that laetrile was not yet an officially approved treatment there. My Mexican acquaintances tell me that a letter explaining laetrile's legal status was sent in 1977 by the incoming administration of President José Luis Portillo.

(The details on the so-called Mexican 'banning' of laetrile are sketchy. I gleaned the above facts by reviewing a May 2, 1977 debate that *NBC News* anchor Tom Brokaw, and science writer Frank Field, moderated between Daniel Martin and the laetrile proponent, Michael Culbert.)

It was characteristic of Martin, however, to inflate a boilerplate letter from the Mexican government into a grandiose story of a negative clinical trial, with unsubstantiated "evidence" of his own devising.

How to Detect Metastases

B
efore launching into a detailed consideration of the laetrile tests at Sloan-Kettering, we must first take up what might seem an obscure topic: how best to detect lung metastases in experimental animals. As the reader will discover, the issue is anything but trivial. In fact, it lies at the heart of the entire question of laetrile's effectiveness in the SKI experiments. Without understanding this question, one cannot understand how Sloan-Kettering was able to state with even the slightest degree of plausibility that Sugiura's results with laetrile were in error.

A metastasis, or secondary growth, originates as a single abnormal cell that typically migrates through the blood or lymphatic system to a distant organ, where it establishes a new tumor. While primary cancers, such as of the breast, may be painful and disfiguring, they do not usually kill their host and they can usually be removed through surgery. It is cancer's ability to travel silently from a primary site to a vital organ that actually kills around 90 percent of the people who die of cancer.[131] Controlling metastases is thus one of the most urgent questions in cancer research.

This fact explains why Sugiura's findings with laetrile were so important. Very few agents, then or now, have been conspicuously effective at controlling the spread of cancer. So even though it is true that Sugiura's experiments were only performed in lab animals, they pointed to the possibility that laetrile (a drug that in all the SKI experiments was non-toxic when injected properly) might be one of those rare agents that could significantly inhibit the deadly spread of the disease.

All of the authors who contributed to the final SKI paper on the testing of laetrile in mice with spontaneous tumors used various combinations of three basic methods for detecting the presence of metastases.

The basis of SKI's criticism of Dr. Sugiura was that he used an intrinsically flawed methodology, whereas those who claimed to have negative results used more accurate methods. It was SKI that drew a sharp distinction between Sugiura's allegedly 'defective' methodology and their own allegedly more accurate ways of detecting metastases.

They were right that one methodology was definitely superior, while the other methodology was spurious, inaccurate and erroneous, and has fallen by the wayside in laboratories all over the world. So let us see which of the competing methodologies was indeed more accurate, and which one has been properly discarded.

Sugiura's Techniques

Sugiura's techniques were simple. At the conclusion of the experiment, he would 'sacrifice' (kill) the animals (or let them die a natural death) and then visually inspect their lungs. He would begin by making naked eye observations, supplemented with use of a magnifying lens. In science this is called a "gross" or "macroscopic" observation. The SKI paper's authors invented a unique term, "macrovisual," to describe these techniques. (Although this word appears nowhere but in this single paper, I will follow their phraseology for the sake of consistency.)

Sugiura considered gross or macrovisual observations to be an obligatory first step toward the detection of metastases. But he always sought independent verification of his own macrovisual findings from an independent pathologist, who looked at slides of the same lungs under a light microscope.

A pathologist is a board-certified physician who has received postdoctoral training to look for, and characterize, malignant cells by their appearance and growth pattern under the microscope. (Today pathologists also extensively use other tests, such as for cell surface markers typical of particular cancers.) Pathologists deal with mouse tissue much as they do human surgical specimens that have been sent to them for identification. In other words, after making a gross examination, they finely slice suspect tissue on a device called a microtome, affix these specimens to glass slides and scrutinize these specimens under various powers of the microscope. This is called a histologic examination.

The SKI paper identifies five pathologists who participated in the laetrile study. The senior one was Myron R. Melamed, MD (1927-2013), a famous figure in cancer pathology. The co-author of over 500 peer-reviewed articles, he is remembered as a co-inventor of flow cytometry.[132] From 1979 to 1989

Melamed was chairman of the MSKCC pathology department.[133] The four other pathologists involved in the laetrile study were Drs. Mohammed Badruz Zaman, K. Komuro, H. Sato and N. Imamura.

When Sugiura and the MSKCC pathologists looked at lungs in this sequence, laetrile was found to profoundly inhibit the spread of cancer from the breasts to the lungs of the mice. On the other hand, inert saline solution (sterile salt water) yielded no inhibitory effect, but on the contrary allowed metastases to develop in a high percentage of test animals.

Now let us look at the competing methods. In the negative laetrile experiments, most of the scientists also looked at the animals' lungs with their naked eyes. For two of Sugiura's challengers, Drs. Elisabeth Stockert and Franz Schmid, that was considered a sufficient examination and their study ended there. On the other hand, Dr. Daniel S. Martin, in his later experiments, substituted a novel technique called a bioassay. (which I shall discuss at greater length below). In his hands, this technique revealed no significant difference between treated and control mice.

That is the crux of the dispute between these scientists. Just to be clear, Sugiura used a macrovisual examination followed by an independent pathologist's microscopic examination, Stockert and Schmid used a macrovisual examination alone, while Martin substituted his exclusive bioassay for the pathologist's exam. Sometimes (as we shall see) Martin skipped macrovisual observations entirely and went straight to the bioassay.

The SKI paper accurately highlighted the discrepancy between these various diagnostic techniques, but then whole-heartedly embraced Martin's method, while it disparaged the techniques utilized by Sugiura. In fact, one could say that SKI staked everything on the superiority of the unusual method of Dr. Martin.

Let us therefore look more closely at the three methods—macrovisual, microscopic and bioassay—to see which were in fact dependable, and which were not.

Critique of the Macrovisual Method

The SKI paper correctly points out that the macrovisual method is only accurate in a rough way. Gross or "eyeball" observations are useful in identifying suspicious abnormalities that might turn out to be metastatic cancer. However, the paper correctly states that macrovisual observations alone might overlook smaller, atypical or less immediately apparent growths, or might mistake non-cancerous tissue for malignancy. So, the paper says, using the macrovisual method alone is frowned upon in any study that aspires to scientific certitude. The paper emphatically criticizes this method when it is used alone. The SKI authors assertively state:

> "*Gross visual observations of the lungs are subjective determinations and may vary with the observer.... These subjective differences in perception of incidence of metastases can make the all-important difference on reporting the experiment as either positive or negative as regards the effect of laetrile upon the spread of cancer to the lungs*" (p. 91).

And again:

> "*The macrovisual [observation, ed.] may not be sufficiently sensitive and also has the possibility of subjectivity in non-blind experiments*" (p. 118).

This is true. But the weird thing here is that the SKI authors (by whom we mean primarily Stock and Martin) were making this point in order to falsely accuse Sugiura of relying on the macrovisual method. It must therefore be stated with equal force that Sugiura did not consider a macrovisual examination sufficient unto itself. He always complemented his macrovisual observations by engaging the services of the MSKCC pathologists who were cooperating in the laetrile project.

In Sugiura's laetrile studies, there was always a high degree of concordance between his macrovisual observations and the microscopic observations of the pathologists.

Thus, overall, the SKI paper itself shows that in the first six CD8F1 treatment experiments, Sugiura saw metastases in the lungs of 48 out of 55 control animals, or 87.3 percent. MSKCC pathologists saw metastases in 41 out of the same 55 control mice, or 74.5 percent.

In the laetrile-treated mice, Sugiura macrovisually saw metastases in 16 out of 90, or 17.8 percent, while the pathologists saw metastases in 16 out of 72 (some mice being held back for bioassays), which constituted 22.2 percent.

The reader can see at a glance the high degree of agreement between Sugiura's visual determinations and those of the pathologists.

Let us look in greater detail at one typical experiment, CD8F1 treatment experiment #2 (summarized on p. 94 of the SKI paper). Sugiura saw lung metastases in 8 out of 10 control animals, while the pathologist saw metastases in 7 out of 10. In only one animal (the mouse designated #1) did Sugiura report metastases in the lungs while the pathologist did not. In the laetrile-treated group Sugiura saw metastases in none of the 10 treated animals, whereas the pathologist detected metastases in a single mouse.

The final SKI paper does not comment on the significance of the general agreement between Sugiura's findings and those of the pathologists. I therefore asked Joseph M. Mahoney, PhD, a professor of engineering with a background in statistics, to analyze the numbers in the SKI laetrile paper and to prepare a report for me on the significance of these and other statistics.

(Prof. Mahoney only provided numerical results from his statistical analysis of the data but disavows any medical inferences for the results. The views, claims, and arguments expressed in this book are not necessarily those of Prof. Mahoney.)

Comparing the conclusions of the MSKCC pathologists with those of Dr. Sugiura, Mahoney confirmed the general agreement of their results. He analyzed the animals that were assessed by both, and restricted himself to those in which the pathologists used microscopy. Using a standard statistical tool called a one-tailed McNemar's test with exact binomial calculations, Prof. Mahoney concluded that "overall there was no significant difference in how the two researchers identified metastases." In other words, there was a significant agreement between Sugiura and the MSKCC pathologists.

In some experiments, SKI used bioassays instead of microscopic examinations. But even when one adds in these bioassays there was still agreement between Sugiura's visual observations and those of the pathologist.
Mahoney comments,

> *"This suggests that overall there was no significant difference*
> *in how the two researchers identified metastases."*

In fact, gross observation, followed by a professional microscopic examination of suspicious tissues, has been in wide-scale use for over a century.
For decades, Sugiura employed, improved and taught this combination of
macrovisual and histological methods to doctors and graduate students.

MSKCC was and is proud of its pathology department and
doctors and patients from all over the world consult it for
highly accurate determinations of suspect tissue. At its Web
site, MSKCC states that its pathologists "see a greater percentage of unusual
tumor specimens in a week than most pathologists see in a year."[135] So a
basic researcher such as Sugiura could not have hoped for a better "reality
check" on his macrovisual observations than the pathologists who coop-
erated in the laetrile experiments. And, as I have shown, these pathologists
confirmed his macrovisual observations.

Yet, amazingly, the SKI paper ascribed the exclusive use of the macrovisual technique to Sugiura. In the Addendum to the SKI paper it states that
Sugiura "employed primarily a macrovisual or subjective method to determine his evidence for laetrile activity on metastases" (p. 112).

This is highly misleading. Sugiura did use macrovisual methods, but
even a glance at the columns of data in the SKI paper reveals that he never
depended on the macrovisual method alone. He supplemented this with
the independent judgment of the pathologists.

This criticism of exclusive reliance on the macrovisual method actually
needed to be directed at two other SKI scientists, Dr. Elisabeth Stockert
and Dr. Franz Schmid, who in their independent experiments *did* rely
exclusively on gross or macrovisual observations. They then used these
"eyeball" observations to contradict the histologically verified observations
of Sugiura!

As the SKI final paper states:

> *"Consequent experiments independently by Stockert and by*
> *Schmid also failed to confirm Sugiura's initial observations"*
> *(p. 121).*

Two Tables in the SKI paper summarize the experiments of Stockert (p. 99) and Schmid (p. 101). These show the percentages of test mice that developed lung metastases. I shall deal with the actual numbers in a moment. But my point here is that these charts were clearly based entirely on Stockert and Schmid's *macrovisual* observations. At the same time, the paper's commentary on these tests fails to inform the reader that these authors' negative conclusions were based on "subjective" macrovisual observations that are excoriated elsewhere in the paper and erroneously ascribed to Sugiura.

To summarize, the SKI paper identified a method of limited accuracy (i.e., the exclusive reliance on macrovisual observations) but then *reversed the record* of who depended on this method and who incorporated more accurate supplemental methods of detection. Stockert's and Schmid's subjective observations were then used in an attempt to undermine Sugiura's objectively verified findings.

The reader can confirm the accuracy of this observation by accessing the SKI paper itself at the Web site of the publisher, Wiley.

Such a clumsy and transparent deception by Sloan-Kettering's leaders should have set off alarm bells throughout the scientific community, first and foremost with the SKI Scientific Advisory Board, which had prime responsibility for detecting misconduct at the Institute. This failure can largely be ascribed to the Nobelist Sir Peter Medawar, a charming man and delightful essayist who, by his own admission, lacked the "moral courage" to expose the misdeeds of senior colleagues whom he had pledged to oversee.[136]

At the May 1977 SKI press conference, Sugiura attempted to refute the blatant distortion of his methods. Here is what he said:

> *"Gross examination of metastases is very difficult. Therefore*
> *everybody should make microscopic examination of the*
> *lungs...I did."*

At the conference, an employee group to which I belonged called *Second Opinion* (to be described in greater detail below) distributed a *Special Bulletin* with questions for the paper's authors. Question #7 was directed to Dr. Stockert:

> *"Why did you not ask the Pathology Department to confirm your gross visual impressions of the mice's lungs with the microscope, as Dr. Sugiura did? How can you say you 'duplicated' Dr. Sugiura's experiment, if you didn't?"*

There was no answer from her or from the SKI administration.

If there is another instance of such outright flouting of obvious facts in a scientific paper, I am unaware of it.

Imagine for a moment that such a transparent deception had been perpetrated in *support* of laetrile. A great many scientists would have reacted quickly. In fact, something like this happened that very year. In 1977, the chairman of the biology department at Loyola University of Chicago, Harold W. Manner, PhD (1926-1986) announced highly positive results against cancer in mice with a combination of pancreatic enzymes, vitamin A and laetrile.[137]

There was "considerable skepticism among scientists elsewhere who have seen his findings," wrote the *New York Times*.[138] Chief among these, the *Times* revealed, was none other than C. Chester Stock!

The Bioassay

At their press conference, and in the final laetrile paper, SKI leaders strongly advocated use of Daniel Martin's "bioassay" as a substitute for both macrovisual and histological examinations of tissues. What was this bioassay, about which Martin and his SKI coauthors waxed so enthusiastic?

Although Martin, as a surgeon, would have routinely employed the services of pathologists, in the mid-1970s he invented a technique that he claimed eliminated the need for a pathologist's examination of suspect tissue for cancer. Martin's bioassay did not rely on any visual observation of metastases, either grossly or with the help of a microscope. In the 1974 paper that introduced the bioassay, he described this new technique as follows:

"The entire lungs from each mouse were carefully minced and divided into portions, [which] were then implanted into the left and right axillary regions of two recipient male mice.

"Subsequently, the test mice were palpated weekly for the appearance of tumor in the region of the axillary implant. The test was considered positive for the presence of lung metastasis if a tumor developed in at least one of the sites of bioassay implantation."[139]

To put this more plainly, after suspect tissue was injected into a recipient mouse, the primary method for determining the presence of metastases was by feeling with one's fingers for the swelling characteristic of a tumor.

In this original paper, Martin continued:

"The lung growths were confirmed as metastases of the mammary adenocarcinomas [breast cancer, ed.] by histological [microscopic, ed.] examination. In every instance, positive and negative results were confirmed by dissection and gross inspection of the axillary site of the implant following sacrifice of the test mice."[140]

But there is a problem here. This may have been how the test was originally conceived, but it was emphatically not how the test was carried out in the laetrile studies. We know this based both on what the SKI paper says about the test procedure and what Sugiura told me and others at the time the test was being performed.

Here is how the bioassay is described in the SKI paper. Notice the subtle departure from the description of the test given in the earlier paper:

"[In a] bioassay for detection of pulmonary metastases—all of the lungs of each animal are shredded…and injected subcutaneously into 2 male CD8F1 mice…If a tumor subsequently arises at an injection site, it indicates that cancer cells (at least 10^5 cells) were present in the lungs."

There is no mention here of utilizing the services of a pathologist to perform a "histological examination." Since, in Martin's view, there was "no subjective element" in his bioassay, he dropped the need for confirmation by an independent pathologist before declaring a subsequent swelling to be metastatic cancer. In fact, the whole point of his bioassay was to eliminate the expensive services of pathologists.

Sugiura told me that he saw no sign that such examinations took place at Martin's laboratory. In fact, it would have been impossible for Martin to perform both a bioassay and a thorough microscopic study on the same mouse, since both required the entire lungs of the animal in question. Otherwise, how could one know that cancer was not lurking in the portions of the lung that were being withheld for one or another of the tests?

The SKI paper was unstinting in its praises of the bioassay:

> *"It is clear that the bioassay represents a more sensitive method of evaluation for metastatic cells" (p. 113).*

But clear to whom? No one else had adopted the bioassay. The paper was simply reiterating Martin's self-serving opinion on the superiority of his bioassay, not presenting facts derived from experimental data. It was not "clear" at the time, and is much less clear today, that the bioassay could replace the tried-and-true methods used by Sugiura and everybody else in the field of experimental cancer research.

In fact, this scientific paper at times adopted a hucksterish tone when addressing the topic of the bioassay. One would have thought that Stock and especially Good would have avoided this sort of error in the wake of the Summerlin Affair. But Stock, as first author, had provided each author a great deal of latitude over his or her "own" section of the paper, and Martin especially took advantage of this latitude to promote his bioassay. This was after all the bioassay's one moment of notoriety, and Martin intended to make the most of it.

If one took the laetrile paper at face value, Sloan-Kettering's top leaders were abandoning decades of successful use of the tried-and-true methods and advocating this entirely unproven method in its place.

But the real reason for adopting and promoting the bioassay was that its use led to conclusions that undermined Sugiura's positive findings.

> *"It is significant that bioassay was the criterion employed in the majority of the negative experiments, whereas, in contrast bioassay was little utilized in the so-called positive experiments" (p. 91).*

It is grimly amusing to see SKI leaders digging themselves deeper and deeper into a hole as they enthuse over the superiority of Martin's bioassay. Taking this position required them to severely criticize the normal methods of histology. They finally went so far as to claim that a typical pathology exam was flawed and insufficient. The reason?

> *"Only portions of the lungs are observed microscopically. Thus the choice of those portions sent for microscopic assay is, like the macrovisual method, a subjective decision...an area of metastasis may be missed" (p. 91).*[142]

"No subjective element," indeed! Without getting into a discussion of the philosophy of science, the idea that one can readily eliminate all subjectivity from any branch of science is at best naïve.[143,144] One should in fact be suspicious of any scientist who tells you that there is "no subjective element" in his or her methodology. No single branch of knowledge can lay a claim to total objectivity.[145]

The SKI authors used repetition to drive home the supposed superiority of Martin's bioassay.[146] They called it "the objective and more sensitive method" and "the only objective method of evaluation" compared to either macrovisual or microscopic examination. They waxed eloquent:

> *"Bioassay is more sensitive and totally objective than the other 2 methods, which have a large subjective element present (p. 91).*

The SKI authors denigrate as subjective a skilled pathologist's use of the microscope:

> *"In the relatively small numbers of animals per group per experiment such differences could make for either statistical*

significance or insignificance. Thus, the subjective element
present in either the macro- or micro-method of detecting
metastases, can allow for a positive experiment (i.e., an
apparent demonstration of anticancer activity), or a negative
experiment (i.e., an apparent lack of anticancer activity"
(p. 91).

This only refers to hypothetical situations, not to what actually happened in any of Sugiura's experiments. In reality, as my consultant Prof. Mahoney has calculated, both the macroscopic observations of Sugiura and the microscopic methods of the independent pathologists produced statistically concordant results. This is immediately apparent when one consults the SKI paper's own tabulated data. So there was little reason to fear that in practice these methods would yield grossly inaccurate results, and in fact there was no particular need to improve on them.

What the SKI paper failed to explain is that surgical pathologists, who are tasked on a daily basis with characterizing human tissue specimens, face exactly the same problem. In the real world, a surgeon removes a specimen for further analysis and sends it to a pathologist in a nearby laboratory. The pathologist freezes a portion of tissue for rapid analysis, and chooses other portions to be preserved in paraffin wax for a more detailed subsequent analysis. This was, and remains, the basic technique that doctors around the world use to decide whether or not to operate on a patient. Everything ultimately depends on the "subjective" decision of pathologists. We rely for our very lives on the skill, knowledge and wisdom of these experts, which is why these "doctors' doctors"[147] go to school for so many years, and apprentice with more experienced colleagues, in order to reach a high degree of expertise.

Ironically, Martin's "day job" was as a surgeon. So in his daily work he too necessarily relied on the very methods that he and Stock excoriated in the SKI paper.

Of course, it is praiseworthy to want to improve tried-and-true methods. But it verges on the delusional to suggest that a method you invented just a few years before, untried in every other laboratory in the world, could suddenly substitute for methods that had stood the test of time for almost a century.

Given Martin's desperate circumstances at Catholic Medical Center, combined with his "enthusiastic" personality (to quote Stock), it is no surprise that he seized upon the SKI paper as a last desperate chance to advertise his method to the world. What is shocking is that sober SKI authors lent themselves to this debacle. Ordinarily, a cautious person such as Chester Stock would never have endorsed such an untested and idiosyncratic method. But politics makes for strange bedfellows, and laetrile was certainly entangled in medical politics at the highest level.

The World Standard

How can the reader be sure that Sugiura's method was indeed the world standard, whereas Martin's method represented a drastic and untested departure from the norm?

A review of the journal *Cancer Research* (publication of the American Association for Cancer Research) for the years 1976-1977 revealed that every article that dealt with the question of rodent metastases used some variant of Sugiura's methods.[148,149,150,151,152,153,154]

Only a single study utilized the bioassay, and that, not surprisingly, was by Daniel Martin and his group. At MSKCC, other researchers in 1977 utilized techniques that were similar to those used by Sugiura. For example, after a macrovisual observation of the animal, the neurologist Jerome B. Posner, MD, and other MSKCC authors wrote:

> *"Histological sections were prepared from each block of tissue and stained.... In several animals, histological sections were prepared from the vertebral column, spinal cord, lung and liver."*[155]

'Histological' means the microscopic examination of tissue. Sometimes the microscope would reveal the presence of metastases that were not visible to the naked eye, or it might fail to confirm the malignant nature of a cellular anomaly. The microscope was therefore seen as an essential adjunct, which is why Sugiura always made use of it.

Modern-Day Use of Bioassay

After publication of the SKI laetrile paper there was no change in medicine's reliance on Sugiura's tried-and-true methods. There was only a gradual refinement of techniques, such as normally occurs in every field. This built upon, but certainly did not repudiate, Sugiura's methods.

Today, papers on the detection of metastases continue to utilize modern-day variants on Sugiura's techniques. In 2012, I searched PubMed (an online index of 23 million biomedical citations) and selected six representative studies of lung metastases in experimental animals. My main criteria for inclusion were that the papers appeared in high-impact scientific journals and were funded by the National Institutes of Health. In other words, I wanted only mainstream articles that were characteristic of contemporary practices.

The 100 or so researchers who co-authored these papers worked at the National Cancer Institute,[156] Harvard University,[157] the University of Rochester,[158] the University of Virginia,[159] the University of Texas M.D. Anderson Cancer Center,[160] the Beatson Institute for Cancer Research,[161] and other top institutions. They can therefore be considered representative scholars of this topic.

Five of these six papers utilized a combination of macrovisual and microscopic techniques to search for metastases, while one used macrovisual observations alone.[162] None used, or even mentioned, any bioassay.

Another way of examining this question is to look at another government database, PubMed Central (PMC), a free full-text archive of 2.9 million biomedical and life sciences journal articles. In the 40 years since Martin introduced his bioassay, only two PMC articles[163,164] have so much as referenced his initial paper on the topic,[165] and neither of these groups adopted the method in question.[166,167]

Nor is Martin's type of bioassay even mentioned at the Web sites of the American Cancer Society (ACS), National Cancer Institute (NCI), American Society of Clinical Oncology (ASCO) or Memorial Sloan-Kettering Cancer Center (MSKCC).

One could justifiably call Martin's technique "defunct," except that might imply that it once had currency in science, but had since lost it. In fact the use of his bioassay for detecting metastases never happened, except in a few papers from Martin's lab and, of course, in this one laetrile paper. In the SKI laetrile paper, Martin's bioassay reached its apotheosis and then, having served its purpose of 'discrediting' Sugiura, disappeared like a stone thrown into the deepest part of the ocean.

It is particularly telling that even SKI's leaders immediately ceased making any further mention of Martin's bioassay. Chester Stock's final scientific paper (1985), which he co-authored with Robert A. Good, also involved a search for metastases. But they conspicuously failed to mention the bioassay, instead writing:

> "*The AK[R] mice already had evidence of leukemia-lymphoma complex in the thymus as revealed by both macroscopic and microscopic criteria.*"[168]

Both 'macroscopic and microscopic criteria'! But weren't those exactly the same two methods that Stock himself had excoriated in the laetrile paper? Of course. Stock continued to use the same methods as Sugiura had used in the laetrile studies, without the slightest comment, explanation or excuse.

He further stated:

> "*Mice which at necropsy [the surgical examination of a dead body, ed.] showed a grossly enlarged thymus and greatly enlarged lymph nodes or spleen were classified as being leukemic.*"

Here also he relied on macrovisual observations, the very method that he and his colleagues blasted Sugiura for using in the SKI laetrile studies.

In the end, even Martin reverted to reliance on Sugiura-type methods. In a February 1977 article (written at about the same time as the laetrile paper) he stated explicitly:

> "*Those lungs with grossly obvious metastatic lesions were not bioassayed.*"[169]

In other words, growths that were visible to the naked eye did not require additional bioassays. This statement was published just a few months before the press conference at which he rebuked Sugiura for failing to use the bioassay on visible metastases![170]

After the appearance of the SKI laetrile paper, Martin published several papers on cancer[171,172,173,174,175] but never again mentioned the bioassay. A 1981 paper offered a lengthy review of adjuvant chemotherapy, but again failed to mention the bioassay.[176] Finally, in a 1992 paper he states:

> *"Patients who had readily accessible tumor tissue...*
> *underwent serial biopsies..."*[177]

But serial biopsies are the microscopic analysis of tissue by surgical pathologists. Once again, there is no mention of the bioassay.

To reiterate, then, other than in the single 1978 SKI laetrile paper, neither Martin, nor Stock, nor Good nor anyone else affiliated with SKI or Catholic Medical Center ever advocated, much less adopted, Martin's bioassay.

This "more sensitive and totally objective" (p. 91) method, which was used to bludgeon laetrile into oblivion, itself quickly dropped from sight.

Nature of the Swellings in Martin's Bioassay

I cannot leave this topic without explaining *why* it was that Martin, using his bioassay, saw little difference between the rates of metastases in laetrile-treated vs. control animals. At the SKI press conference, Sugiura explained the reason for this to the assembled reporters:

> *"But remember, bioassay—you need good experience,*
> *because sometimes tumors keep on growing for two, three or*
> *up to eight weeks. That's adenocarcinoma [the kind of cancer*
> *found in CD8F1 mice, ed.]. But when tumors sometimes*
> *grow for a couple of weeks and then start to regress, that's*
> *not adenocarcinoma. Of course, then you need examination*
> *by microscope. If you look under the microscope, that's not*
> *adenocarcinoma."*

In other words, swellings that arose at the site of a bioassay implant, which Martin claimed represented the rapid development of malignant tumors, were not necessarily cancerous. Sugiura himself had also performed bioassays in some of his experiments. He had some of the subsequent "tumors" analyzed by MSKCC pathologists and these were not actually cancer. They were simply non-malignant inflammatory reactions.

The raw video footage of the SKI press conference is very revealing on this point. Sugiura began to explain Martin's fallacy. Visibly flustered at the imminent exposure of the weaknesses of his method, Martin rudely interrupted his scientific opponent. Addressing the reporters, with a gratuitous swipe at Sugiura's Japanese accent, he said:

> *"If you'll read the paper...I think you'll be better able to*
> *understand what I don't think was well expressed by*
> *Dr. Sugiura here in...ehr... English. The sentences there will*
> *explain some of the things you just think you heard, but I*
> *don't think you heard it right. It's all there in black and*
> *white...if you take the trouble to read the paper. An*
> *unequivocal, biological report to you that laetrile is without*
> *biological activity."*

At the time, Martin's exhortation to "read the paper" brought a smile to my lips since, moments before, Jerry had instructed me to hide copies of the paper in question behind a heavy curtain in an adjoining room, and to only give them out to reporters who explicitly asked for them. Only two did.

Sugiura's point was well taken, though, even if few reporters understood him. If a recipient mouse were injected subcutaneously with another mouse's lung tissue, there would frequently be a swelling at the injection site. But this swelling wasn't necessarily cancerous. It was usually just an inflammatory reaction to the introduction of foreign material.

Sugiura found that one needed to wait eight or nine weeks in order to differentiate between these two fundamentally different types of swelling. If the growth diminished, then the "tumor" was not dangerous, much less fatal. But if you sacrificed the mouse after detecting a swelling of any type at the implantation site, as Martin hastened to do, and did not bother to have an independent pathologist examine those tissues under the microscope, then you might erroneously conclude that the mouse's lung was positive for cancer.

This was the major source of false positive test scores on Martin's bioassay. Martin was seriously over-diagnosing cancer in the lungs of treated animals by designating temporary inflammations as deadly tumors. Since this occurred equally in laetrile-treated and control mice, there then did not appear to be any significant difference between the two.

The problem of "false positives" in bioassays was well known at the time. For instance, a type of bioassay was in use at the National Toxicology Program (NTP) of the National Cancer Institute. In 1977, just before the SKI paper was released, the statistician David S. Salsburg, PhD, had estimated that the false positive rate in these bioassays was between 20 and 50 percent.[178] In a 2008 re-analysis, it was shown that many of the results in these bioassays were false positives.[179]

So the unreliability of bioassays was well known. Any attentive reader of the scientific literature knew about it. Yet, with their backs to the wall over the laetrile issue, Sloan-Kettering's leaders enthusiastically endorsed Martin's test, thereby dooming laetrile, but also discrediting the reputation of their institution.

Sugiura's Laetrile Experiments

I shall now trace the progression of Sloan-Kettering's mouse experiments with laetrile, from the first experiments in spontaneous tumors in the summer of 1972 until final publication of their paper in the *Journal of Surgical Oncology* in February 1978.

My primary sources are the two slightly different versions of the SKI paper: the preliminary version that was released at the June 1977 press conference and the final paper published (with an Addendum) eight months later.

I have supplemented these with Sugiura's meticulous laboratory notes, a copy of which he gave me on May 6, 1975, and which were later reprinted in the Committee for Freedom of Choice pamphlet, *Anatomy of a Cover-up.*[180] These notes correlate well with the paper. In the end, Stock did not tamper with the raw data because its accurate publication was Sugiura's requirement for participating in the June 1977 press conference.

In 1972, Lloyd Old had written to clinicians who were using laetrile, asking whether they believed it to have any value in the treatment of human cancer and, if so, which types. He asked detailed questions about routes of administration, dosages employed, and how rapidly one might expect to see a response. He also asked, "Why has there been so much controversy surrounding the use and effectiveness of laetrile?"

The responses he received were of a mixed nature and "not consistent," he said. But one common observation was that laetrile eased pain. Anecdotally, some laetrile-using patients claimed that they were able to give up mind-clouding narcotics, as well as experience an increase in well-being and appetite.

In mid-1972, Sloan-Kettering convened a meeting of the "Therapy Field" to affirm an institution-wide decision to proceed with laetrile testing. Stock, predictably, proposed testing laetrile in transplantable tumor systems that were widely in use at that time.[181] Typically, cancer-free animals were injected with small tumors or with a carcinogen, and then a proposed treatment was administered to destroy this tumor. There had been previous tests elsewhere of laetrile in such systems and these had failed to find any significant activity. These included a dozen different transplanted experimental tumors. There was no reason to expect it to perform any differently at SKI. Stock anticipated a quick study of, perhaps, a few months' duration and a rapid answer for Benno Schmidt.

Indeed, Sloan-Kettering quickly confirmed the work of other groups that laetrile failed to have any anticancer effect in transplantable tumor systems.[182] Many people were relieved that the world's premiere cancer center had confirmed what others had been saying for decades: laetrile didn't work. (Results of these studies were published simultaneously with the more controversial results on spontaneous tumors.[183])

But at that time there was a growing feeling that transplanted tumors were too artificial a system in which to achieve results that were predictive for human cancer. In 1973, *Science* stated that "there are many scientists who are beginning to question the virtue" of transplanted tumor systems. It summarized their opinion that:

> "...transplanted tumors may be quite unlike natural or
> spontaneous ones, that they may possess special enzyme
> systems which control their response to chemical agents, and
> that they may be anything but representative of tumors in
> man."[184]

Humans, for example, do not normally have tens of millions of cancer cells suddenly thrust upon them in a single implantation. A tumor naturally originates as a wayward cell, which grows and metastasizes from an initial point of development, in constant struggle against the host's immune system. In fact, with a few conspicuous exceptions, transplantable systems had failed to find many agents that were effective against the "garden variety" of solid tumors of adults; this was taken as proof of their artificiality.[185]

Even NCI recognized that "the selection of the appropriate experimental model [was] critical to cancer drug discovery and development."[186] So Old was hardly alone in believing that spontaneous solid tumors were the most promising way of testing new compounds.

Spontaneous tumors, arising in the course of an animal's unhampered development, are a more true-to-life model. But mice with spontaneous cancer take 8 or 10 months for visible tumors to appear. During that time one has to feed, cage and otherwise maintain them. They were comparatively expensive and, once a palpable tumor had appeared, much more difficult to cure.[187]

But in the summer of 1972, SKI made the fateful decision to extend laetrile testing to mice that spontaneously developed tumors. The scientist who was asked to perform these tests was Kanematsu Sugiura, DSc, the Institute's oldest and most experienced researcher. Testing rats and mice with cancer had been his forte for over half a century. Another reason he was chosen was that he had long been retired (although he continued to work every day). Thus, if the tests came under unfriendly scrutiny, SKI could rightly say that no donor's money had been expended testing a "quack" remedy.

First Sugiura Experiments

From the start, Sugiura's experiments achieved highly positive findings. Laetrile, he told Stock and Old, worked in a number of interesting ways, most significantly in its ability to stop the spread of cancer. Filled with what Stock later called "scientific caution," they asked Sugiura to repeat his experiment. No one had ever asked Sugiura to repeat an experiment before, in fact he was famous for getting things right the first time. But naturally he complied. Increasing the dose to 2,000 milligrams per kilogram of body weight, he got even better results. Amazed, Stock asked him to repeat the test again. And again. And again. Six treatment experiments in CD8F1 mice. Then they asked him to repeat the test using a different method of evaluating metastases. Then with a different source of laetrile. Then in different animal systems. Between September 1972 and February 1975 Sugiura performed a total of nine tests in three different systems: laetrile came out positive, in very similar ways, in all of these tests. It temporarily stopped the growth of small tumors, shrank cancerous organs, improved the animals' health and well being, and stopped the spread of metastases in mice. It was not a cure for cancer, he said, but "a good palliative drug."

He was understating the case. By 1974 it was clear that laetrile had a greater efficacy at stopping the spread of cancer (particularly, lung metastases) in mice than any other agent then known.

Summary of Laetrile Results

In the summer of 1974, in the course of my interview for MSKCC's *Center News*, Sugiura told me:

> "Laetrile can't work on transplantable tumors. When I use it on a large spontaneous mammary [breast, ed.] tumor like this"—he made a circle with his thumb and forefinger about the size of a dime—"it has no effect. But a small tumor like this"—he made a tiny circle—"about one centimeter in diameter, laetrile stops the growth. Not permanently, but for a week, two weeks, three weeks....
>
> "The most interesting part," he continued, "is metastases. When this mammary tumor grows to about 2 centimeters in diameter or more, about 80 percent develop lung metastases. But with treatment with amygdalin, it's cut down to about 20 percent."

Metastases are secondary growths that migrate from the primary tumor and invade other areas of the body. Such secondary growths are often more lethal than the original tumor.

I was of course astonished at what he was telling me. "With all these positive results, why is there all this controversy?" I asked Sugiura.

"Many people still doubt my work, and so I show them all my work in this book—you see," and he took down from the shelf above him a volume, one in a long, uniform set of laboratory books, going back decades. "I keep records like this," he said, thumbing through the pages. "Here, amygdalin—."

The emeritus scientist pointed to pictures of small mice, each with an irregular circle on its breast—the outline of a tumor. The pictures were made with a rubber stamp that Sugiura had used for decades. (He had worn out a few.) He stamped the outline of a generic mouse and then drew not only the size of a tumor but its location on the body.

In addition, Sugiura said, laetrile-treated mice definitely seemed healthier and friskier than the salt water or saline-treated control mice. That spring, with millions of others, I had seen the *60 Minutes* segment on laetrile and I read of patients who claimed pain relief with the treatment. What Sugiura was saying about "healthier and friskier" results seemed similar to anecdotal reports of pain relief filtering across the border from Tijuana, Mexico. I asked Sugiura what he thought of these reports. He added quickly:

> *"I think there must be some benefit. Dr. Old believes it. I think most people in this institution don't believe my work, although I show them results like this."*

He laughed sadly. I then asked the senior researcher if he had published any of these results.

"No, not yet." He hesitated, and then said, "I'd like to, but it's up to the people downtown." In Walker Lab parlance, "downtown" meant SKI headquarters on 68th St. in Manhattan. "Dr. Old, Dr. Stock, if they want to publish it, they'll publish it."

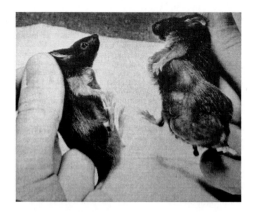

Martin's CD8F1 mice

I got the feeling it would never have occurred to him to publish the results independently. Scientists today generally work as part of a team and one needs the "permission" of the team leader to submit such work for publication. In fact, in January 1976, Sugiura submitted a completed paper on his nine laetrile experiments to his immediate supervisor, Stock. But Stock declined to publish this independently, although most of the data did eventually appear in the final paper two years later.

"Are you still doing work on amygdalin?" I asked him.

"Oh yes, I'm now doing work on prevention. In the first experiments [i.e., the first CD8F1 treatment experiments, ed.] the mice already had tumors, see? But in the latest experiment the mice have no tumors. At four months old, with no tumors, I started to inject amygdalin to see whether or not mammary cancer develops. These are strains of mice that are sure to get cancer in about 80 to 85 percent of the cases, during a lifetime of from two to two and a half years. Now it's eighteen months and we've gone through three-quarters of their life span, and I have found that the controls, receiving only saline injections, developed cancer in fifteen out of thirty cases. But the experimental animals, receiving laetrile, have developed only six tumors out of thirty mice, or about 20 percent."

In a massive understatement he added:

> *"It would be interesting if it prevented it completely. One*
> *hundred percent prevention would be very interesting—then*
> *it would convince everybody. I never heard of anybody trying*
> *to repeat my experiment. Somebody should repeat my work.*
> *Not from this institution, somewhere else, a different*
> *institution."*

Sugiura then drew a parallel between his own difficulties and those of William B. Coley, MD, whom he had known at Memorial Hospital for two decades.

"Nowadays, natural things are coming back more and more," Sugiura said. "Dr. Coley was working before 1900 with toxins prepared from bacteria. Doctors used to laugh at Coley as 'nonsense.' Now it's no longer nonsense. Bacterial toxins contain polysaccharides, which inhibit the growth of tumors in animals. Japanese scientists are finding that polysac-charides prepared from mushrooms can destroy tumors in mice."[188]

He went on (referring to laetrile by its technical name, amygdalin):

> *"Amygdalin, too—people now are laughing at that, especially*
> *the director of the National Cancer Institute and the*
> *American Cancer Society. They even wrote a book,*
> Unproven Methods of Cancer Management, *with chapters*
> *on Coley's toxins, laetrile, and so forth."*

"Why are they so much against it?" I asked Sugiura.

"I don't know," he said, hesitating. "Maybe the medical profession doesn't like it because they are making too much money."

Unconscious Bias?

I found Sugiura to be perfectly lucid. In fact, this mental acuity was why SKI asked him to test laetrile in the first place. In my conversations with him he always displayed a comprehensive awareness of both the details and the overall situation. His memos and reports on the progress of the experiments were clear, factual and exceptionally well written.

But in its final paper SKI made the charge that Sugiura was "uncon-sciously biased" in his evaluation of laetrile. One does not normally criti-cize one's colleagues in print, much less in papers containing their own results. And make no mistake: conscious or unconscious bias are fighting words in science, as "bias" of any kind is among the most damning things one can say about a colleague.

This was particularly strange since no one could recall a single other instance in 60 years in which Sugiura had shown the slightest bias in either his personal or professional life. As a Japanese-American in World War II he may at times have been the victim of bias, but there is no record that he ever reciprocated. So the idea that Dr. Sugiura had suddenly developed a bias in favor of some notorious "quack" remedy from California seemed highly implausible. In fact to people who knew him it was a laughable absurdity.

His "unconscious bias" was never defined, but presumably meant that while he may have intended to be objective, he was so strongly predisposed to find laetrile effective that he translated that into the creation of numerous false reports sent to his superiors.

It was bizarre in the extreme to hear Daniel Martin, a man who had an undisguised and obsessive hatred of laetrile, accuse the even-tempered Sugiura of being biased in his assessment of the same substance!

Not surprisingly, the accusation of "bias" rested on a gigantic and deliberate misreading of the facts. After enumerating Sugiura's consistent findings of benefit in his first six experiments, the SKI paper stated:

> "It is possible for the investigator (who employed primarily a macrovisual or subjective method to determine his evidence for laetrile activity on metastases) to be unknowingly biased in his subjective readings by his knowledge of which animals were in the laetrile-treated group" (p.123).

So here, once again, was the oft-repeated falsehood that Sugiura employed a purely macrovisual way of determining the presence of metastases. Elsewhere in this book I have exposed the falsity of this claim. As I have shown, Sugiura not only examined lungs with his eyes and with a magnifying glass but fully utilized the services of MSKCC pathologists, who provided independent verification of his macrovisual observations. This is shown unambiguously in the data Tables of the SKI paper itself.

Since Sugiura, whenever allowed to do so, always had his results double-checked by MSKCC pathologists, even had he been a laetrile fanatic, which he emphatically was not, it would have been impossible for him to influence a single pathologist's judgment. As I also show elsewhere in this book, Sugiura's macrovisual observations and those of the pathologists generally agreed quite well. They each arrived at their evaluation of metastases in the lungs by different methods, but their shared conclusion was that laetrile stopped the spread of cancer to the lungs of treated animals.

In other words, Sugiura did not have the "means, motive or opportunity" to influence the independent testimony of five MSKCC pathologists, or to induce them to corroborate his supposedly falsified observations.

There was no plausible way in which both Sugiura and these skilled pathologists could be simultaneously incorrect in their determination of lung metastases. So SKI had to find some other explanation for Sugiura's and the pathologists' conclusions that laetrile was a highly active agent.

This is what ultimately led them, in an act of desperation, to attack the methods not just of Sugiura, but of their own pathology department. These were time-tested microscopic techniques. They realized that to agree to the accuracy of these standard methods would invariably lead to a confirmation of the objectivity of Sugiura's laetrile findings.

We are thus treated to one of the weirdest spectacles in the history of cancer research, in which top scientists, including Lewis Thomas, Robert Good and Chester Stock, suddenly became implacable critics of the very methods that they themselves and their institution normally relied upon. By adding their names and reputations to this laetrile report, they were endorsing the idea that the commonly used macrovisual and microscopic methods were fundamentally flawed, and that this flaw had therefore yielded false positive results for laetrile.

Once things had quieted down, all three of them (along with everyone else in science, including Daniel Martin) went back to their unquestioning reliance on the normal methods, without mentioning that they ever thought otherwise.

We can thus conclude that the sweeping attack on the combined macrovisual and microscopic methods in the SKI paper was never meant to be a serious critique, but was merely a temporary measure adopted to discredit Sugiura's positive findings with laetrile.

Sugiura's CD8F1 Treatment Experiments

We now come to a closer examination of the six treatment experiments that are at the core of the controversy. These were carried out in mice that spontaneously developed mammary, or breast, cancer. This mouse was designated CD8F1 (more precisely CD_8F_1) and was developed by Dr. Daniel S. Martin in the late 1950s when he crossed two mice strains that spontaneously developed breast cancer. In the 1970s, his breeding colony in Queens, NY was the sole source of these mice.

As Lloyd Old later explained to *Science,* one's choice of a testing system was and is crucial in determining the outcome of an investigation:

"Old explains that the model system in which chemicals are
evaluated is important and may partially explain why he
and his colleagues are seeing some activity [with laetrile,
ed.], whereas other investigators (other than committed
laetrile scientists) have found none."[189]

In other words, a drug could fail in various evaluative systems and then, suddenly, work in another. This is not exactly a "contradiction." Sugiura was using a relatively new mouse model and looking for an unusual parameter of benefit, the reduction in lung metastases.

On September 12, 1972, he began his first experiment with "amygdalin MF" (supplied by the McNaughton Foundation) in CD8F1 mice. Four months later, in January 1973, he reported his results in writing to the top SKI administrators. Laetrile, he told them, was not a cancer cure (a popular myth), but it did have other significant effects:

- Laetrile stopped the spread of cancer to the lungs of the animals;

- It temporarily stopped the growth of small primary tumors by about three-quarters; and

- It improved their general health and well being.

But Sugiura always made clear that laetrile did not shrink, much less cure, primary tumors. He therefore classified it as a good palliative drug. The lack of curability should not have been a total surprise, since many laetrile proponents avoided the word "cure," claiming instead that the drug was a means of control. Author Glenn Kittler, for instance, had originally titled his book, *Laetrile: Control for Cancer.*

How had so many other scientists missed this fact in the past? Part of the reason was that Sugiura was working with rare and expensive spontaneous tumors, as opposed to those that involved transplanted tumor tissue. Another reason was that Sugiura looked at the lungs of the animals for signs of cancer's spread. Untreated, it turned out that these mice developed metastases in a high proportion of cases. Laetrile greatly diminished their occurrence. By 10 months of age, when their primary tumors averaged one gram in weight, about 80 percent of them had developed lung metastases.[190]

In an internal memo to the administration (later quoted in *Science*), Sugiura wrote:

> *"The results clearly show that amygdalin significantly inhibits the appearance of lung metastases in mice bearing spontaneous mammary tumors and increases significantly the inhibition of the growth of the primary tumors over the appearance of inhibition in the untreated animals."*[191]

One would think that scientists all over the world would have reacted to these findings with utter elation. After all, drugs to treat metastatic spread were (and are) rare. But this was not to be the case. To understand the shock that this report caused, you must remember that this was the first time that any well-regarded institution had reported positive effects of any kind with laetrile. American cancer experts had spoken with an increasing degree of certainty about the ineffectiveness of laetrile. It was almost universally believed to be a "quack remedy." And there was absolute confidence that the world of therapeutics could be neatly divided between "approved" and "unapproved" treatments, the latter of which were virtually synonymous with quackery.

But if Sugiura's observations were accurate, then an entire generation of American scientists had been wrong about laetrile. Dead wrong. It was not a "quack remedy," the bogeyman conjured up by that watchman of medical morals, the Unproven Methods Committee of the American Cancer Society. Nor was it the "vitamin B17 cure" of popular legend. It was, in Sugiura's words, simply "a good palliative drug." This was a modest claim, but to accept it required a complete philosophical shift on the part of those who divided the cancer world between "proven" and "unproven" methods, and were sure that they could divine the difference between the two. So naturally there was consternation when word of Sugiura's results started to leak out of Sloan-Kettering.

Happily, we know a great deal about Sugiura's experiments because he was a meticulous record keeper. All of Sugiura's six CD8F1 treatment experiments followed the same pattern. According to his notes:

- *Every* mouse in *every* experiment was numbered individually. Mice were "earmarked" through the placement of a hole, notch or double notch in one or both ears.

- Both the initial and the final size of its tumors were measured in millimeters.

- The average size of these tumors was calculated.

- The duration of each experiment was noted for each mouse and averages were given.

- There was an observation of the effect of treatment on the growth of the primary tumor, including any inhibition in growth.

- Finally, there was a description of the extent of lung metastases. Sugiura gave a rough indication of how many metastases he saw in the lungs. This was then double-checked by an MSKCC pathologist.

The SKI paper later summarized Sugiura's first six studies with CD8F1 mice:

> "In a series of 6 experiments with CD8F1 mice with
> spontaneous mammary adenocarcinomas [breast cancer,
> ed.], Sugiura noted...an overall average of 21 percent of mice
> with lung metastases... compared with 90 percent of the
> control mice" (p. 89).

I asked my statistical consultant, Prof. Mahoney, for his analysis of this portion of the experiments. On Sugiura's set of experiments he stated as follows:

> "This suggests a significant difference in the probability of
> metastases between the control and treated cohorts. The
> relative risk (RR) of metastases was 0.206. Thus, an animal
> in the treated group was about a fifth as likely to have a
> metastasis as an animal in the control group."

In these experiments, there was a visible difference between the lungs of the treated animals and the controls. For example, by Sugiura's observations all of the lungs of the animals in the second experiment were free of cancer, whereas 80 percent of those in the control group had lung metastases.

Sugiura also found that laetrile had a positive impact on quality of life. As Sugiura put it in the SKI paper:

> *"All mice with large tumors appeared in better health in the treated group compared with similar controls" (p. 92).*

Prophylaxis Experiment in CD8F1

In addition to the six treatment experiments in CD8F1 mice with established tumors, there was a single prophylaxis (prevention) experiment (SKI paper, pp. 100 and 102-103). This was conducted over a period of two-and-a-half years. During this time Sugiura injected and examined each mouse seven days per week, never taking a break or a vacation. Unlike Martin, Sugiura never utilized lower-status lab assistants to do the day-to-day work of injecting, tending or evaluating the animals. He was a hands-on scientist of the old school.

In this prevention experiment, there was no significant difference between the two groups in terms of primary tumor development. However, there was a difference in metastases. My statistical consultant calculated this as significant (using a Chi-square test). The relative risk (RR) was 0.3125. This means that a laetrile-treated mouse had roughly one-third the chance of developing metastases as a control mouse.

Prevention of metastases is the key to controlling cancer, since metastases kill 90 percent of people who die of cancer. So, if these results held in human clinical trials this could have been one of the most important findings in the history of cancer research. To this day, I can find nothing that quite equals it. The closest I have seen was a 2005 study of the drug taxol and the dietary supplement curcumin (from turmeric root) in a nude mouse model.[193]

How did SKI deal with a 79 percent decrease in the appearance of lung metastases? To diminish its significance, they simply lied about the manner in which it was achieved. In the pre-print that was the subject of the June 1977 Press Conference, they wrote:

"The difference in lung metastases was evaluated only by macrovisual observation."

This was untrue. The difference between treated and controlled animals was evaluated by both macrovisual and microscopic examinations by MSKCC pathologists. We know this because the data in the paper itself tells us so.

One of the most astonishing things about this astonishing paper was the brazenness with which they repeated this lie in the face of the data in their own Tables! There is really no way to appreciate their nerve except by comparing their statements to the data given in the paper itself. It was breathtaking in its arrogance.

Here is how the SKI authors concluded their description of the prevention experiment:

"Our findings now reveal otherwise in a clinically therapeutically-relevent [sic] animal tumor model. Moreover, laetrile's effect upon the development of spontanteous [sic] mammary cancer in CD8F1 mice was tested by Sugiura in a prophylaxis experiment …and the findings were negative with respect to the prevention of cancer."

This is a blatant falsification of the actual results of Sugiura's prevention experiment.

Sugiura's AKR Leukemia Experiments

A second system in which Sugiura tested laetrile is called the AKR mouse. Prof. Jacob Furth of Cornell University, New York, had created this mouse 40 years earlier[194] through the intensive crossbreeding of three separate strains.[195] AKR mice developed leukemia spontaneously in 60-90 percent of cases, with a peak incidence at eight months of age. According to a 1973 paper by Lloyd Old, "the importance of the AKR mouse strain in leukemia research is widely recognized."[196]

In these mice dying of leukemia, Sugiura saw no preventive effect from laetrile and the effect on survival was also negligible (pp. 104-105 and 110-111).

However, Sugiura wrote in a July 25, 1975 memo that there was an important and potentially beneficial effect on the internal organs: on average, the size of the thymuses was reduced by 50 percent, of involved lymph nodes by 45 percent and of spleens by 25 percent. The thymuses of the laetrile-treated animals had a median weight of 75 milligrams (mg) whereas the weight of the thymuses in the control animals was 351 mg, or more than four times as large. Overall, this constituted a large decrease in the weight of the leukemic thymuses. My statistical consultant tried to analyze this but found that the paper did not include the organ weights per animal. Without this, he was unable to determine whether or not there was a significant difference between the two cohorts.

According to Sugiura's memo of May 17, 1975, laetrile "prevented the enlargement of lymph nodes in AKR mice—approximately 50 percent...."[197]

Laetrile, he said, "had a certain inhibitory action on the development of leukemia in mice....[Laetrile] is not a cancer cure but a good palliative drug," he repeated.[198,199]

The shrinkage of organs and glands involved in immunity was ordinarily taken as a sign of anticancer activity in this system. For instance, Lloyd Old's group had reported in 1973 on the destruction of leukemia cells in AKR mice by immunological means (other than laetrile).[200] In those experiments, shrinkage of lymph nodes and spleens was taken as a sign of an anti-leukemic effect in AKR mice.

Robert A. Good was a world expert on the thymus and so these facts were certainly well known to him. A 1970 study, by SKI's Robert Kassel, had noted that interferon treatment reduced the size of the thymus in leukemic animals (although they were still two to three times normal size).[201]

An article by SKI researchers Kassel, William Hardy and Noorbibi K. Day made clear that shrinkage of lymphatic tissue greater than 20 percent was a sign of anti-cancer activity. They specified inguinal, mesenteric and cervical lymph nodes and spleen.[202]

While more than the 20 percent benchmark was reached in the case of the laetrile-treated animals' thymuses, this fact was never mentioned in the SKI paper. Here is how the SKI paper summarized Sugiura's AKR findings:

> *"Amygdalin at 2,000 mg/kg/day was ineffective both in treating and preventing the development of spontaneous leukemia in AKR mice."*[203]

("Mg/kg/day" was scientific shorthand for "milligrams of drug per kilogram of body weight per day.")

This was only half-true, since the paper failed to tell us what of a positive nature was achieved in this study. Other experiments with AKR leukemia pointed to the significance of diminishing the size of the thymuses. For instance, a more recent study from Suzuka University of Medical Science, Japan, studied the effect of a botanical extract on the incidence of leukemia in AKR mice. They found that the mean weight of the thymuses of control animals was 219.9 mg, compared to 145.0 mg in treated animals.[204] They called the increase in thymic weight "markedly suppressed"[205] by the administration of this agent. This worked out to a 34.1 percent decrease, which was less than Sugiura saw with laetrile.

I therefore conclude that Sugiura observed some positive effects with laetrile in AKR leukemia, but SKI chose to obscure that by drawing sweepingly negative conclusions in the comment section.

Sugiura's Swiss Albino Experiments

A third model was the Swiss Albino mouse obtained as a retired breeder from Taconic Farms, Inc. of Germantown, New York. These animals normally developed spontaneous breast tumors in about 60-70 percent of cases but were only available in small numbers. As with CD8F1, their primary tumors were also exceptionally difficult to cure. According to the SKI laetrile paper smaller tumors stopped growing temporarily in 24 percent of controls and 52 percent of laetrile-treated animals. While 91 percent of the control group showed lung metastases by visual observation, only 22 percent in the laetrile-treated mice did so. Also, the general health and appearance of the laetrile-treated mice seemed better than the corresponding controls (p. 104, see also pp. 107-108).

Thus, there was a 28 percent absolute decrease in tumor progression, and an astonishing 69 percent absolute decrease in lung metastases. I can find no record of any similarly positive numbers with any non-toxic therapeutic agent. But in their commentary, rather than acknowledging his success, the SKI administration leveled criticisms at Sugiura's results:

> *"Although this experiment was not subjected to an appropriate independent trial and no bioassays of the lungs were made, it is included in order to present all of our properly completed anti-tumor tests" (p. 104).*

The "General Discussion" of the SKI Paper also claims that the reduction of lung metastases in the treated mice "had not been subjected to the challenge of independent confirmation."

But if Sugiura's critics did not perform any confirmatory experiments in this animal model, one can hardly fault him for this. The decision to do, or not do, a confirmatory trial in Swiss Albino mice was out of his hands, and in the hands of the very people who later made this criticism.

Let us parse these charges one by one.

The SKI paper states that "[t]he results must be looked at questionably… in the light of the paucity of information on metastases in Swiss mice, the lack of bioassays and in view of the lack of confirmation of Sugiura's metastasis studies in CD8F1 mice."

I would answer these charges as follows:

- Sugiura was very familiar with Swiss Albino mice and in fact he and Stock together had performed studies in this mouse as early as 1950.[206,207] In 1956 Sugiura published a study that included a determination of lung metastases in these mice.[208] It was only two decades later, after Sugiura had achieved highly positive results with laetrile in these mice, that Stock disavowed the results because of Sugiura's supposed lack of prior experience with this system.[209]

- A lack of concordance with Martin's bioassay would only be a deficit if this were recognized as a truly superior method for detecting lung metastases. But, as I show elsewhere in this book, it most emphatically was not. So this is a meaningless charge.

- The supposed "lack of confirmation" of Sugiura Swiss Albino results in CD8F1 mice is bizarre. Even if, for the sake of argument, we were to grant laetrile's supposed "ineffectiveness" in CD8F1 mice, how would that negate the possibility that it could be effective in Swiss Albino mice? The variability of responses from system to system is the principal reason that most potential anti-cancer agents are tested against a spectrum of models, and not just a single one.

Sugiura's positive results in Swiss Albino mice were strikingly similar to those in CD8F1. In both kinds of mice, laetrile greatly inhibited the growth of lung tumors and improved health and well-being. The arguments that SKI advanced to obscure this fact are specious. Nowhere does the report state in clear, unequivocal terms that Sugiura's Swiss Albino studies confirmed his positive findings concerning lung metastases in CD8F1 mice, but that is indeed what happened.

Effect Upon Cells

We might note here that Sugiura, who trained with "the Chief," James Ewing, MD in the histologic examination of cancer cells, tried to answer what was occurring at the cellular level in animals receiving laetrile. After a microscopic examination of the animals' tumors, Sugiura noted:

> "There were many mitotic figures among the control tumor cells while tumor cells of amygdalin-treated animals appeared more hemorrhagic, degenerated, and contained fewer mitotic figures."[210]

The appearance of "mitotic figures" is a sign of active malignancy, while the presence of hemorrhage (bleeding) and degeneration is a sign that something is killing those cells. Sugiura made similar observations in the lymph nodes of AKR leukemic mice, but these important observations were omitted from the report and never mentioned again.

Reaction to Sugiura's Experiments

S tarting in the late fall of 1972 there was considerable agitation at SKI over Sugiura's positive findings. Some people were energized, but for most people at SKI, Sugiura had obtained "what might in one perspective be called the 'wrong results'," wrote Nicholas Wade in *Science*. Stock in particular was worried. "Normal scientific caution," he later said, demanded that other scientists repeat Sugiura's results.

The Laetrile Task Force

Lloyd Old took Sugiura's positive results as a signal to expand the testing of this, as well as other, non-conventional or "unproven" methods.

"At the Memorial Sloan-Kettering Cancer Center on the upper east side of Manhattan," wrote Barbara J. Culliton in *Science*, "some perfectly respectable scientists are taking a look at some thoroughly unrespectable cancer remedies."[211] Old told *Science*,

> *"One can always look at unproved methods for possible leads."*[212]

It is hard to realize how provocative this statement was to the "quack-buster" mentality, which was so prevalent at the ACS, FDA and elsewhere.

I later obtained from Lloyd H. Schloen, PhD, a postdoctoral student in Old's laboratory, the minutes of an internal meeting of a newly formed "Laetrile Task Force," dated July 10, 1973. These minutes showed the following in attendance on the thirteenth floor of the Howard Building: in addition to the top three SKI officials, Good, Stock and Old, there was Raymond Brown, MD; Dean Burk, PhD; Ernesto Contreras, MD; and Dr. Contreras's physician son.

Also in attendance were Raymond Ewell, PhD, the retired vice president for research of University of Buffalo; Andrew McNaughton, the Canadian sponsor of the laetrile movement; Mrs. Helen Coley Nauts; and Morton K. Schwartz, PhD, a biochemist who worked with Old on many projects.

Contreras's presence deserves special mention, since for over three decades he was a key figure in the laetrile story. He was responsible for treating thousands of individuals in Tijuana, including the first American laetrile patient, Ms. Cecile Hoffman, who later founded the International Association of Cancer Victims and Friends.

Contreras was much maligned in the US media. But he was a graduate of the Mexican Army Medical School (Escuela Medico Militar), which has been called "a prestigious source of military medical physicians for the Mexican armed forces."[213] He had served as the chief pathologist at the Army Hospital in Mexico City and was also a Professor of Histology and Pathology at the Mexican Army Medical School. In the 1940s he did postgraduate work at Children's Hospital, Boston, a Harvard-affiliated institution.

It is noteworthy that Old assumed the honesty of his guests and did not seem fazed by the fact that some of these individuals were described by many of his own colleagues as "cancer quacks." Never before had so many proponents of alternative medicine been included in a high-level meeting at Sloan-Kettering or, one suspects, at any other American scientific institution.[214] It would take another 20 years for the National Institutes of Health to gather a comparable group in Chantilly, Virginia, to lay the groundwork for what is now the National Center for Complementary and Alternative Medicine.

During this same period, advocates of other unorthodox approaches, such as Virginia Livingston, MD and Eleanor Alexander-Jackson, PhD (proponent of bacteria as a cause of cancer), Joseph Gold, MD (advocate of a metabolic agent, hydrazine sulfate), Karl Ransberger, PhD (co-developer of the German enzyme supplement, Wobe Mugos), and Hans Nieper, MD (German clinician and formulator of laetrile derivatives) were also invited to top level meetings at Sloan-Kettering.

The First Leak

In September 1973, Sugiura's confidential memo, "A Summary of the Effects of Amygdalin (Laetrile) Upon Spontaneous Mammary Tumors in Mice," was leaked and sent to the attorney for John A. Richardson, MD. The latter was an Albany, California doctor who was on trial for administering laetrile to patients.[215] Nobody ever took responsibility for the leak. Most likely, these notes fell into the hands of one of the individuals attending the "Laetrile Task Force" meetings at SKI, who sent them to Richardson's attorney, George W. Kell. He shared a copy with reporter Harry Nelson, who in October 1973 published an article on them in the *Los Angeles Times*.

Nelson later recalled his mixed emotions upon receiving Sugiura's memo to the SKI administration:

> "As I read the full report I felt both elated and depressed. The elation was because I realized that I had the first evidence that I had ever seen by a reputable researcher that laetrile may be something more than a hoax. The depression came even before I had verified with SKI that the report was not a fake. I realized that if I wrote the story there would be a helluva uproar from the medical establishment, and if I decided not to write I would have to answer to myself for suppressing what appeared to be legitimate news."[192]

This honest assessment encapsulated the ambivalent feelings of many reporters (and scientists) who approached the question with any degree of objectivity.

SKI Visits Baden-Baden

Undeterred by the brouhaha over the document leak, Old sent Dr. Lloyd H. Schloen and an older associate, Raymond Brown, MD, to two important meetings.

The first was the Congress of the International Medical Society for Blood and Tumorous Diseases in Germany. This evolved into "Medicine Week" (*Medizinische Woche*), which is still held every October in Baden-Baden. In 1973, cancer researchers and clinicians from more than 15 countries attended.[216]

Raymond Keith Brown (1922-2013) was a soft-spoken family doctor from the eastern shore of Virginia, who, in his small clinic, had revived the use of Coley's toxins. This brought him to the attention of Mrs. Nauts. In 1973 he moved to New York City and became a Cancer Research

Institute Fellow at Sloan-Kettering. For a while he served as a sort of pleni-potentiary from Sloan-Kettering to the CAM community.

About 600 health professionals listened in rapt silence as Schloen detailed Sloan-Kettering's initial success with laetrile. Dean Burk, PhD, the most prominent advocate of laetrile at the National Cancer Institute, accompanied Schloen and Brown. He later told me that Schloen's state-ment was a watered-down version of his original text:

> "*Every hour on the hour [Schloen] was getting telephone calls from Sloan-Kettering to keep taking this out and that out. There wasn't too much left when he got through.*"[217]

But enthusiasm for laetrile at Sloan-Kettering kept mounting throughout 1973, in parallel with Sugiura's positive findings. In April, SKI sent Schloen and Brown to the first annual convention of the International Association of Cancer Victims and Friends (IACVF), the pro-laetrile organization headed by Ms. Cecile Hoffman.[218]

Laetrile seemed about to break out of the unorthodox "ghetto" into which it had been consigned for the previous two decades and to become a respectable treatment. In fact, the age-old divide between "orthodox" and "unorthodox" cancer treatments itself seemed to be dissolving rapidly.

Science *Article*

In December 1973 Barbara J. Culliton wrote in *Science* about Dr. Good's open-minded attitude toward the testing of unorthodox methods, including laetrile. Following the leak, the MSKCC Public Affairs Depart-ment drew up a cautious statement for distribution:

> "*The Sugiura report is preliminary and part of a broad ongoing scientific inquiry. It would be premature at this time to draw specific conclusions on the basis of the Sugiura report.*"[219]

The Public Affairs Department, Culliton wrote, was:

> "*...fully aware of the large laetrile cult in this country and of the fact that desperate cancer patients will try anything.*

*They did not want to put the prestige of their name behind a
drug they were light-years from endorsing, because they
knew the harm that it could do."[220]*

Science endorsed Sloan-Kettering's positive, but cautious, approach to
laetrile:

*"The fact that the institute is paying serious attention to
laetrile and other unorthodox ideas which, it thinks, have
just enough of a shred of truth to make them worth a second
look, is something many people see as a step ahead for
science."[221]*

The Holleb Letter

Initially, Robert A. Good, MD, PhD, Director of Sloan-Kettering Institute, had expressed trust in Sugiura's skill and therefore in his laetrile
results. He told *Science*:

*"I think from everything we know that he [Sugiura, ed.] is a
reliable scientist, and he has an extraordinary record
through the years of being right."[222]*

But soon the first cracks appeared in this sensible approach. Good was
under enormous pressure, both from without and within SKI. There is
documentary evidence of this pressure campaign.

Patrick Michael McGrady, Jr. (1932-2003), son of the science editor of
the American Cancer Society, unearthed the most important piece of
evidence. In the course of researching an article on a German cancer
clinic,[223] the younger McGrady gained access to off-limits files at ACS
headquarters. Pat was a charming fellow who cajoled one of the secretaries
into letting him consult the confidential files. Before ACS officials knew
what was happening, he had copied a confidential letter and reprinted it in
the April 1976 *Esquire*.

The letter, dated January 1974, was from ACS's Chief Medical Officer
Arthur Holleb, MD (1921-2006), who had transitioned from a Memorial
Hospital breast surgeon to the leading paid employee and most powerful

executive of the ACS.[224] In this letter, Holleb wrote to SKI President Good expressing his dismay at Sloan-Kettering's new open-minded posture toward alternative treatments.

Here is what Holleb wrote:

> *"I wish I knew how one could better control the unfortunate and premature publicity which links my distinguished alma mater to the promotional side of these unproven methods. We have both agreed that the public will be best served if tests are properly conducted in a prestigious institution, but the exploitation of the good name of the Sloan-Kettering Institute is becoming embarrassing. Perhaps your staff would be willing to consult with us and review our files before commitments are made."*[225]

In a world filled with diplomatic and coded missives, this was strong language indeed. 'Unfortunate,' 'promotional,' 'exploitation' and 'embarrassing' were not words one usually used when addressing the president of the nation's most important cancer institute, a man who was second only to Benno Schmidt in the hierarchy of the "war on cancer." But we have to understand that ACS 'fed' Sloan-Kettering and not the other way around.

ACS contributed almost $4 million a year to Memorial Sloan-Kettering at a time when the Center was suffering from what officials called a "disquieting deficit of $5 million" due to "expansion of research programs for which funding was simply not available."[226] Everyone knew that Good had run up these deficits in his expansion of the immunology program. ACS could either help remedy that situation or make it much, much worse.

Immediately, Good altered both the tone and content of his public statements about laetrile. In December 1973, he had told *Science* that there was evidence "on both sides of the fence" on laetrile. But on January 10, 1974, he declared:

> *"At this moment there is no evidence that laetrile has any effect on cancer."*[227]

No evidence? Good had already received a formal report on Sugiura's first three positive experiments in CD8F1 mice. In addition, SKI (in the person of Lloyd Old) had received the technician Shelly Jacob's memo on her positive experiment with Swiss Albino mice.

A few months later Good would join Old, Stock and Thomas at FDA headquarters in Maryland to present Sugiura's results in a favorable light and plead for the right to do clinical trials with laetrile. So if there was truly "no evidence that laetrile has any effect on cancer," as Good said in January, then why would he join this high-level trip to the FDA in July, taking a day out of his busy schedule to plead on the drug's behalf?

What he said in January 1974 was politically expedient, but was simply not true.

In the 1973 *Science* interview, Good complained that he was being subjected to a "pressure cooker" atmosphere around the topic of laetrile, which subverted the "natural processes of science." Following the "natural processes," however, Sugiura would have simply published his positive results, and then others could then have published their own results, positive or negative.

Good was in a nightmarish situation. He already knew that outside scientists were unable to reproduce his and Summerlin's claims in the transplantation project. Huge deficits were looming as he tried to implement expensive programs. And now the laetrile problem had fallen squarely in his lap. His brief tenure at SKI was imperiled, and his long-sought goal, a Nobel Prize, was slipping from his grasp.

So, on January 10, 1974, with his "no evidence" statement, Good became the first SKI official to lie about the outcome of the Institute's laetrile experiments. He simply denied the existence of Sugiura's positive tests.

Throughout my employment at MSKCC I too encountered the intense hostility of some medical leaders towards laetrile. One anecdote will suffice. I was having lunch with a TV reporter at a restaurant that was frequented by people doing business with MSKCC. I was talking, perhaps a bit too unguardedly, to this reporter about our laetrile experience. The next thing I knew a portly middle-aged man, visibly intoxicated, approached my table and, without any preliminaries, started shouting at me.

"When are you people at Sloan-Kettering going to stop fooling around with laetrile?" he demanded. "You're an embarrassment to the rest of us."

I was staggered by this unanticipated attack and shamed at being upbraided in front of a reporter. I demanded that the drunken man identify himself. His business card revealed that he was deputy director of the New York office of the Food and Drug Administration! So if I, an anonymous MSKCC employee, could receive that sort of verbal abuse from a government official, I can only imagine the kind of pressure that Good and other Sloan-Kettering leaders were experiencing from higher level officials.

In January, in an interview with Ron Kotulak of the *Chicago Tribune,* Good expounded his new line:

> *"The first tests with the compound [laetrile, ed.] in animals indicated that it might have some anti-cancer effect but subsequent experiments failed to confirm it."*[228]

The Public Affairs Department was also on the spot. On March 15, 1974 Jerry Delaney released this statement on behalf of the administration:

> *"At this time, we have no information that amygdalin is useful in the treatment of human cancer."*

This, technically speaking, was not untrue, because SKI was testing laetrile in mice, not humans. Sugiura's mouse experiments contained no information that was directly relevant to humans. So SKI was misdirecting the debate in a way that many readers might not even notice.[229]

Starting in January 1974, all of those forces that, since 1953, had been pontificating on the worthlessness of laetrile recovered from their shock at Sugiura's results and mustered their forces. They began a campaign to convince Sloan-Kettering's leaders that "all kind of havoc" (to use Stock's phrase) would follow if SKI dared to publish a positive report on laetrile. SKI leaders started to backtrack in public, making increasingly false statements to the media. This became outright lying as the months progressed. To be clear, SKI leaders were not themselves the source of the opposition; but they fell in line with the prejudices of their peers.

For example, after Sugiura's results became well known, Frank Rauscher, PhD, the director of the National Cancer Institute (NCI), told Mike Wallace of *60 Minutes:*

"I would certainly not turn off laetrile if it had an iota of activity that we could pinpoint. Unfortunately, there's no evidence at all."

In January 1974, Charles Moertel, MD, of the Mayo Clinic chimed in:

"Extensive animal tumor studies conducted independently at ...New York Memorial Sloan-Kettering [sic]...have shown this drug to be totally without evidence of anticancer activity."[230]

On March 24, 1974, FDA Commissioner Alexander M. Schmidt (no relation to Benno Schmidt), made a presentation at the American Cancer Society's Science Writers' Seminar. He said the following:

"The Food and Drug Administration is against use of the drug [laetrile, ed.] because there is 'no shred of evidence' that it has any effectiveness at all, he said. 'We have tracked down every lead we could to uncover some evidence of efficacy,' Schmidt said. 'To date we have not found any.'"[231]

"Every study to date has not found any evidence of efficacy. We will not allow trials in humans unless there is some evidence in animal systems that it has biological effect" and only if "our requirements for any IND were met."[232]

What were these requirements?

"One shred of evidence in animal or cell systems of efficacy."[233]

Schmidt lacked one shred of evidence that laetrile worked! Yet Sugiura's positive experiments had been fully described in Barbara Culliton's *Science* article in 1973, and everyone in science read *Science*. So unless these distinguished medical leaders (Schmidt, Moertel and Rauscher) were living in caves, they had to know that Sugiura had already provided not just a shred but a wealth of evidence of laetrile's effectiveness against metastases. Yet with no fear of contradiction from SKI, these top administrators confidently put forward the exact opposite of the facts.

At the moment that these medical leaders were saying such things in public, Sloan-Kettering's top officials were privately trying to arrange a laetrile clinical trial with their counterparts at the 20th of November Hospital in Mexico City. They had to plan such a trial in Mexico because the FDA, as a matter of policy, had frustrated every attempt to perform a trial in the United States.[234]

Soon after he sent his momentous letter to Good, Holleb emerged as the *de facto* spokesman on Sloan-Kettering's laetrile experiments. That's right, the ACS vice president became the spokesperson on laetrile for SKI! The immediate effect was to twist Sugiura's results to remove the slightest implication of benefit from laetrile. Here is how Holleb re-interpreted Sugiura's results for the Associated Press:

> *"An initial report from a scientist at Sloan-Kettering Institute for Cancer Research in New York that laetrile showed some action against cancer cells in the test tube has had no confirmation from later work."*[235]

In the test tube? Was Holleb ignorant of how the SKI animal tests had been conducted? Or was he spreading misinformation to hide the fact that Sugiura had achieved overwhelmingly positive results in mice? To repeat, at this point, there had been six positive experiments in CD8F1 mice and one successful prevention experiment. There were similarly positive results in Swiss Albino and AKR leukemia. So Holleb was in every respect wrong. Sugiura's work had not been refuted. The data was still overwhelmingly positive. Yet with his menacing letter to Good, Holleb had accomplished his goal. He had frightened Good and the other top MSKCC leaders into conformity with the "party line" on laetrile.

Meeting at FDA

In private, at least, MSKCC's leaders attempted to fight back. The growing disparity between the statements emanating from the FDA and the positive results from SKI demanded a resolution. SKI leaders proceeded on the assumption that FDA was unaware of what had actually transpired in Sugiura's tests. So, on the afternoon of July 2, 1974, a meeting on laetrile was convened at FDA headquarters in Beltsville, Maryland.

We are very fortunate that an FDA employee, Howard L. Walker, MD, took minutes, and that these, along with those of an NCI meeting the following year, have survived the ravages of time.

(The fate of these minutes has been a saga in itself. In 1978, Dean Burk, PhD and I testified about laetrile before a committee of the Michigan House of Representatives. John T. Kelsey, the Democratic representative who was sponsoring a bill to legalize laetrile, obtained copies of the FDA and NCI minutes through a Freedom of Information Act (FOIA) request. He then provided me with a copy. After I finished *The Cancer Syndrome* in 1980, a University of California librarian, Robert F. Lewis, approached me to donate my papers to a "Special Collection on Laetriles" at UCSD. Years later, when I tried to retrieve these papers I learned that Mr. Lewis had passed away and that none of his colleagues knew where this "Permanent Collection" might be. When I came to write this book I obtained a fresh copy of these minutes from the Bentley Historical Library of the University of Michigan, where Rep. Kelsey had deposited his papers.)

With these notes, we have a window into the candid thinking on laetrile of top health officials at that time.

The four top MSKCC scientists were in attendance—Robert A. Good, Lloyd Old, Chester Stock and Lewis Thomas. In addition, a dozen leaders of the FDA and NCI were in attendance. They included Bayard H. Morrison III, Stephen K. Carter and Robert M. Hadsell from the NCI and J. Richard Crout and other members of FDA's Division of Oncology Products.

This was a high-powered group. Walker's hand-written notes reveal the confidential thoughts and statements of the leaders of three uniquely powerful institutions, isolated from the scrutiny of the media. In other words, this was not the usual baloney dished out for public consumption, but the inside views of important public figures. One rarely gets to see such a forthright statement of opinions. It is especially revealing for what it tells about the thinking of the four top MSKCC leaders.

Richard Crout and Lewis Thomas (the senior FDA and MSKCC officials, respectively) opened the conclave with general introductions. Then Good reviewed the main scientific questions that he said were of interest to Sloan-Kettering Institute. He emphasized three points:

- "It is hard to identify laetrile as a compound; one can only work with amygdalin;

- "There is immense emotion associated with this drug; and

- "Studies of amygdalin are *a small part* of [the] Sloan-Kettering program."

These platitudes were, nonetheless, true. "Studies on amygdalin" were indeed "a small part of Sloan-Kettering's program." But they happened to be the part that much of the world was intensely interested in and that these top leaders had assembled to discuss. If Good seemed defensive, it was because of criticism that Sloan-Kettering's leaders (to quote *Science*) "had all gone off the deep end because they were studying laetrile and other suspect cancer therapies."[236]

Good told the Rockville group:

> "*The aim today is to present the data to FDA and NCI and to have us think about it.*"

Next, Lloyd Old took over the presentation. Although technically Good's deputy, he had seniority at the Center and had not been implicated in the recent Summerlin scandal. Never comfortable speaking in public, Old confronted a room full of skeptics, most of whom shared a vehement hatred of laetrile and the laetrile movement, to which he had shown some tolerance, if not sympathy. With his typical brilliance, he succinctly reviewed the basic concepts behind laetrile, as it was then understood, including the "selective release of CN (cyanide) intracellularly." He then outlined SKI's ambitious plan to study not just laetrile but related cyanogenic glycosides (such as prunasin). He said:

> "*Sloan-Kettering would like to test these drugs in spontaneous tumors not just experimentally derived tumors.*"

Of course, that program was already underway. He also noted claims that cancer cells had "high glucosidase levels." (This was a popular theory behind laetrile's use.)

Old then recounted his search for clinicians who had actually used the substance. According to the minutes:

> *"Dr. Old has written to several world users of laetrile,*
> *including Drs. Contreras and Niepe[r] and others. He found*
> *two groups: (1) Those who used it and found it of value and*
> *(2) those who had not used it and did not believe in it."*

Old confirmed Sloan-Kettering's findings that laetrile had no effect on transplantable tumors. And then, finally, he came to the nub of the matter. He presented the data, complete with accompanying charts, from Sugiura's repeated studies showing that laetrile inhibited metastases to the lung.[237]

> *"The Sloan-Kettering group believe[s] their results show that*
> *amygdalin used in animals with tumors show: a decrease in*
> *lung metastases; slower tumor growth; and pain relief. The*
> *Sloan-Kettering group are [sic] thinking of a study in man on*
> *pain relief (ibid.).*

As to toxicity in the animal experiments, a major concern of the FDA, the report reads:

> *"Dr. Old feels that amygdalin is as non-toxic as glucose,*
> *although oral administration increases toxicity due to CN*
> *release from bacterial break down."*

He noted correctly that the oral route of administration of amygdalin was more toxic than the injected route "because the intestinal bacteria break down amygdalin to release cyanide." This was a well-known quality of amygdalin that much would be confirmed in the Mayo Clinic human clinical trial.[238]

Laetrile's essential non-toxicity when given by injection was borne out by Sugiura's animal experiments, and most other experiments in which laetrile was injected at the very high milligram-per-kilogram level. Under such circumstances, it had no negative effect on the health of the animals.

Quite the opposite: laetrile-treated animals in a number of experiments seemed healthier.

As to the deaths of some animals in toxicity studies, Old noted:

> *"Deaths following [intraperitoneal, ed.] injections were found to be due to accidental intestinal penetration and action of mouse intestinal bacteria on amygdalin with cyanide release."*

Sloan-Kettering officials explained that they were working with two forms of laetrile: the Mexican version (designated MF, for the McNaughton Foundation) and a German version (manufactured by Sidus Pharma in Munich). The German version, they said, had no effect (an exaggeration), but the Mexican version was active in their experiments.

Old now revealed some data charts from a new "third set" of experiments. Experiments I, II and III are repeats of each other. The results were as follows:

> *"Mexican amygdalin showed an effect in 2/3 experiments. German amygdalin showed no effect. However analysis of slopes showed that both were better than control and Mexican better than German. Both Mexican and German inhibited metastases to the lung."*

"In these comparative tests," Old continued, "there were lung metastases in 83 control animals. 20 German amygdalin treated [and] 18 Mexican amygdalin treated." This is somewhat garbled in the notes, but seems to refer to Sugiura's experiments, which were then ongoing. Next comes a comment with vast implications for a crucial future experiment:

> *"Parenteral [injected, ed.] amygdalin excreted unchanged; oral amygdalin excreted as thiocyanate."*

If injected amygdalin were excreted in an animal's wastes, then it would be present in abundance in the feces and urine of all treated animals. This means that if treated and untreated animals were caged together, they would all share the medicine because they are by nature coprophagic (i.e., eat their own and each others' feces).

This was to become a major issue in the final "blind" laetrile experiment at SKI (see below). Old's summation was as follows:

> *"The Sloan-Kettering group believes their results show that amygdalin used in animals with tumors show: a decrease in lung metastases; slower tumor growth; and pain relief."*

It bears repeating that these were the four top SKI leaders' privately expressed beliefs in March 1974. Yet two months earlier Good had claimed the exact opposite in a newspaper interview.

It is also interesting that in conversation with the FDA, SKI leaders attributed pain relief to laetrile in their animal studies because in his 1973 *Science* interview Good had said that well-being or pain relief "does not show up in animal experiments."[239]

Stock, who was silent throughout most of the meeting, at this point contributed that he "thinks studies on amygdalin should be made particularly regarding pain relief and reduction of lung metastases."

After this buildup at the FDA meeting, the notes rather surprisingly state:

> *"Sloan-Kettering is not enthusiastic about studying amygdalin but would like to study CN [cyanide] releasing drugs."*

In other words, SKI was looking to extend the basic concept of laetrile, as a cyanide releasing pro-drug, to create synthetic compounds that might do the same thing more efficiently. This was probably a result of Old's conversations with the German laetrile specialist, Hans A. Nieper, MD of Hannover, who was creating synthetic spin-offs from amygdalin. One sometimes heard the fear expressed in the laetrile movement that Sloan-Kettering only intended to enrich itself and the pharmaceutical industry and would never use any readily available natural substance. In fairness, we should note that Ernst T. Krebs Jr.'s original idea for laetrile was itself a synthetic version of amygdalin that was supposedly better suited to the enzymatic nature of most cancer cells.

Such drugs could be patented and would have the advantage of more easily fitting under the jurisdiction of the FDA, a point that would hardly need emphasizing in that company.[240]

At the conclusion of the conclave, everything seemed encouraging. The final proposals seemed to indicate that SKI's presentation had been a rousing success:

> *"A discussion ensued on where we should go from here. Agreements:*
>
> *"(a) Sloan-Kettering Institute and NCI will consider clinical trials aimed at treatment of cancer and for the relief of pain and will request consultation with ACS;*
>
> *"(b) There are no regulatory policy problems preventing the study of amygdalin in man;*
>
> *"(c) A standard scientific approach to studying amygdalin is recommended, meaning the drug should be worked up by standard approaches;*
>
> *"(d) FDA will publicly endorse good research on amygdalin as in the public interest."*[241]

These are all extraordinary statements. In almost every particular, they contradicted the official FDA line on laetrile, which was that there should be no clinical trials (for pain or any other indication); that regulatory issues precluded the study of laetrile in humans; and that the FDA discouraged clinical research on laetrile, in fact forbade it on penalty of imprisonment.

Look in particular at this statement:

> *"There are no regulatory policy problems preventing the study of amygdalin in man."*

For 20 years, the FDA had put every imaginable obstacle in the way of studying laetrile in humans, going so far as to aid in the prosecution of laetrile-using doctors, such as John Richardson, MD. In a peculiar twist, in 1970, it had first granted, and then within days rescinded, an Investigative

New Drug (IND) license to the McNaughton Foundation for testing laetrile. Now they were saying (in private) that there was no regulatory obstacle!

In private, FDA and NCI joined SKI in endorsing good research on laetrile "as in the public interest." This was staggering in its implication and the news was never shared with the general public, much less the laetrile movement. The Sloan-Kettering delegation came back to the Upper East Side in an optimistic mood, with a pocketful of empty promises. Theoretically, they had been given a clear path forward that could have resolved the laetrile problem in a brief period of time. But not one of these fine proposals was ever acted upon. It was to be four years before a new director of NCI overturned previous refusals and called for clinical trials aimed at treatment of cancer and the relief of pain.

And, then, it was only because the FDA had identified four trial sites that housed what the contemporary historian Daniel Carpenter, PhD has called "strong laetrile skeptics."[242] The FDA would only allow laetrile to be tested by its avowed enemies, led by the Mayo Clinic chemotherapist, Charles Moertel, MD, whose nickname was "Dr. Debunker."[243]

In the mid-1970s, the FDA did not come out publicly for more research on laetrile; quite the contrary, it maintained its intractable stance that laetrile had been adequately tested for 20 years and was without an iota of value. Nor did the FDA declare publicly that there were no regulatory issues preventing the study of laetrile in humans. Instead it maintained that such studies were both unethical and illegal.

In my opinion, the SKI leaders had been skillfully "played" by the FDA. They went to Rockville in good faith, under the assumption that Commissioner Schmidt had made his negative statements out of ignorance of what had been achieved by SKI. But after they left, nothing changed.

FDA Commissioner Schmidt died in his sleep in 1991, at age 61, so we cannot ask him. But, in my opinion, his misstatements were much more likely the result of calculation than ignorance. He was a skillful Washington insider, who was continuing a "party line" of 20 years duration.

By telling SKI what it had come to hear, however, the FDA, along with the NCI and ACS, bought time. They needed this time to come up with a plausible way of discrediting Sugiura's results and undermining the resolve of SKI leaders to support his work. I shall deal with that momentarily. The short answer to how they accomplished this was Daniel S. Martin, MD.

The Conclave at NCI

Nine months later, on the afternoon of March 4, 1975, a second high-level governmental conclave was held, this one at Building 31, the Claude B. Pepper Building, on the sprawling NIH campus in Bethesda, Maryland. Its purpose was "to decide on what further course of action should be undertaken with this controversial compound." This time, Stephen K. Carter, MD, the Deputy Director of the Division of Cancer Treatment, kept the minutes.

A total of 32 top figures of the War on Cancer were present, including Frank J. Rauscher, PhD, director of the National Cancer Institute; the head of the Division of Cancer Treatment Vincent T. DeVita, Jr. (soon to succeed Rauscher as NCI director); and a dozen of their most powerful subordinates. From MSKCC came Thomas, Old and Stock as well as Edward "Ted" Beattie, head of Memorial Hospital (the clinical arm of MSKCC); Irwin H. Krakoff, a top chemotherapist; and Carl M. Pinsky, MD, an immunologist (and surrogate for the missing Robert A. Good) who later served on Daniel Martin's ASCO Subcommittee on Unproven Methods.[244,245,246] The participation of the surgeon Beattie, the chemotherapist Krakoff and the immunotherapist Pinsky was a show of unity, demonstrating that the laetrile testing program had broader support than just Lloyd Old and his group on SKI's "13 Howard."

Also present on this occasion were Charles G. Moertel, MD, from the Mayo Clinic (who would eventually lead the NCI-sponsored clinical trial of laetrile) and two top quackbusters of the American Cancer Society, Sidney L. Arje, MD, vice president for professional education (whose office published *CA—A Cancer Journal for Clinicians*), and Robert Eyerly, MD, chairman of the ACS's Committee on Unproven Methods. Finally, there was Daniel S. Martin, MD of the Catholic Medical Center.

Carter and Old chaired the meeting, which was opened by NCI director Rauscher. Once again, and, as it turned out, for the last time, SKI's leaders defended Sugiura's laetrile findings. Once again, Old reviewed for them the chemistry of laetrile and its relationship to the other cyanogenic glycosides (CGs). He outlined some of their current research approaches to the CGs and "briefly mentioned the non-toxic nature of amygdalin [laetrile, ed.] in animals." Old summarized the main effects of injectable laetrile in Sugiura's experiments, including of course an average decrease in lung metastases from 80 to 20 percent.

But this time, unlike at the FDA meeting of the previous year, the opposition had found its voice. Martin provided a countervailing interpretation of SKI's test program. According to the notes:

> "Dr. Daniel Martin, of the Catholic Medical Center in
> Queens, New York then briefly summarized his results in the
> CD8F1 mouse system, which is a system he developed and
> with which he has the greatest experience. He has performed
> two experiments with Mexican amygdalin. In the first, the
> amygdalin was given as a suspension and in the second, as a
> solution, which was the way Dr. Sugiura had administered
> the drug. Both experiments were completely negative."

The collaborative study, which Martin and his team had thoroughly botched, had resurfaced as a "completely negative" experiment. I have tried to imagine the emotions of Old and the other SKI leaders as they contemplated this obvious prevarication on Martin's part. However, the notes do not indicate that they contested or confronted this transparent deception.

In the ensuing discussion, two clearly demarcated sides emerged. One side, represented by Old and other SKI leaders, held that "the nontoxic nature of amygdalin made it a superb candidate for a double-blind evaluation." (It was taken for granted in all these discussions that injectable laetrile was nontoxic.) They also said "the preclinical data are [sic] not that critical since the drug is being extensively used." This was clearly backtracking. It is hard to believe that Sugiura's results did not justify a clinical trial, since NCI had nothing comparable to try against metastases.

Another theme, however, was that "the preclinical data, only, clearly do not support a clinical trial being undertaken..." This cannot have been the view of Old, since he had already expressed himself positively on this point.

Recurring point no. 7 was that "there are no convincing clinical data to date," while no. 8 was that "undertaken, a clinical trial in the US would be fraught with many consequences on many levels."

One of the consequences would have been that the FDA, NCI, ACS and other authorities would have had to explain to the public why they were suddenly reversing a verdict on laetrile that had been in place since 1953![247] They could have said simply that new scientific data had emerged, but it is not so clear that the American public (and especially litigious attorneys) would have been quite so understanding on that point.

After three hours of discussion and debate, two choices emerged. The first was to "file an IND and undertake a US trial." The second was to

> *"...visit with Dr. Sannen and help him design an adequate trial in Mexico and observe its progress. A decision on [a] US study would await these results."*

According to the notes:

> *"It was the consensus of the group that there did not exist currently either the clinical or preclinical data to support option I and that option II could lead to that data. It was felt that if the Mexican government would invite NCI to help with this trial, that a group could visit with Dr. Sannen for that purpose and observe the results of any trial undertaken. The group that volunteered to participate included Dr. Charles Moertel, Dr. Irwin Krakoff, and Dr. Stephen Carter."*

In my opinion, it was ludicrous to state that the existing data did not justify a phase I clinical trial in the US. Had SKI's original interpretation of Sugiura's data prevailed, a US trial might have proceeded immediately (instead of one being completed seven years later).

(Given that the focus of this book is on the laetrile experiments at Sloan-Kettering, I am unable to expand here on my views of the NCI-sponsored clinical trial that was published in 1982 in the *New England Journal of Medicine*. I hope at some future date to discuss in print the various deficiencies in that trial.)

What primarily stood in its way was the opposition of Daniel Martin, newly emboldened by his ASCO position and his $1 million grant from the NCI.

Also, the doctors who were selected to oversee a Mexican-based trial were all hard-line chemotherapy advocates. While a Mexican trial would not have to be approved by the FDA, if these three American oncologists were overseeing the testing, there was unlikely to be any positive interpretation of the outcome from the American side. As it turned out, no such Mexican trial was ever performed.

All Out Against Laetrile

One might think that at this point the American cancer establishment would have stopped its relentless assault on laetrile and the laetrile movement. Instead, exactly the opposite happened. There was an upswing in attacks. And, suddenly, Lewis Thomas joined in an intemperate verbal assault against this forbidden fruit pit.

Within weeks of the aforementioned NCI conclave, Thomas appeared before the American Cancer Society's Science Writers' Seminar, which was being held at a San Diego, California resort. At the time, this seminar was a major conduit between the "cancer establishment" and the mainstream media.

At this April 2, 1975 meeting, Thomas gave a new version for public consumption of the results of Sloan-Kettering's testing of laetrile. Laetrile, he now said, had demonstrated:

- No protective effects against cancer;

- A failure to provide any prolongation of life;

- An inability to reduce the size of a tumor; and

- Failure to inhibit the growth of a tumor.[248]

Of course this was an outrageous distortion of what had actually happened and bore no relationship to what SKI leaders had told the NCI, FDA and ACS just one month earlier. These new statements were fabricated to suit the political needs of the moment. The most pressing of these needs was to retain the $4 million in funding that ACS provided MSKCC each year, as well as the various crucial contributions of the NIH and FDA. In *Center News*, the MSKCC Board had already warned employees of a huge budgetary shortfall and that they needed to drastically tighten their belts. For weeks, employees talked of little else. So, financial retribution from major sources of funding at that moment would have been devastating.

However, I was so disturbed by the entirely negative slant of Thomas' interview that I made up my mind to confront each of the top leaders of MSKCC—Good, Old, Stock and Thomas—to learn their rationale for these negative statements.

I asked Jerry Delaney if I could talk to Thomas about his erroneous statements. Naively, I thought he was simply in error and that I might be able to enlighten him about the details of Sugiura's studies. I knew only vaguely about his two trips to Washington to plead for the legitimacy of these studies! Jerry as a matter of territoriality did not like me to see Thomas without himself being present, and he quickly vetoed my idea. But he did promise to ask Thomas for a clarification, and he was good to his word.

A few days later he returned from a meeting with Thomas and, red in the face, relayed something that has stuck with me ever since. He said that Thomas told him:

> *"I am not going to die on the barricades for laetrile. If it were a cure, I might do differently. But it is only a palliative drug."*

I was immediately reminded of Barbara Culliton's humane comment on laetrile in *Science* in 1973:

> *"Even though these effects are not life-saving, to the terminal cancer patient they are anything but inconsequential."*[249]

This particular "palliative drug" also stopped the development of lung metastases in about 80 percent of the CD8F1 mice, an achievement unattainable by any other agent at the time. Thomas' comments struck me as unbelievably cynical and even possibly criminal in nature. Scientific fraud was not then a crime in American jurisprudence and it was to be 30 more years before the first American researcher would go to jail for falsifying research data.[250] But there was no doubt in my mind that the general public was being deceived on a matter of life and death, and apparently there wasn't a thing that I could do about it.

In the newspaper article, Thomas had added:

> *"Details of the study will be published within the next few weeks. He declined details."*[251]

As well he might, since it would be three years, not three weeks, before SKI's twisted version of the laetrile tests would finally be published in the *Journal of Surgical Oncology.*

Just as the ACS's Arthur Holleb had demanded in his letter to Good in January 1974, Sloan-Kettering was now "coordinating" its public statements about laetrile with the masssive ACS publicity machine. Never again would Sloan-Kettering's leaders embarrass their benefactors over laetrile or—to put it plainly—bite the hand that fed them.

I had Thomas' answer but, as part of my plan to personally confront each of the top MSKCC leaders, I made an appointment to see Lloyd Old. When I gingerly raised the topic of laetrile with Old, he asked me, rhetorically, "Do you want to know where we get all our new ideas?"

Of course I did!

He closed the door to his office, walked around the couch where I was sitting, to the built-in wooden bookshelves that lined the wall behind us, and took down a loose-leaf volume.

"Here," he said, "This is our Bible. This is where we get our new ideas." It was the American Cancer Society's *Unproven Methods in Cancer Management*—the notorious quack list!

I had inherited a well-worn copy of this same book from my predecessor, but hadn't given it much attention. The ACS sent tens of thousands of copies of this book to doctors and other opinion makers to guide them away from fraudulent or worthless treatments. However, when (at Old's urging) I studied this list, I realized that the evidence marshaled against these treatments was often very flimsy. This was a blacklist rather than a serious scientific evaluation and, having lived through the McCarthy era and seen its effects, I was not a big fan of blacklists.

One month after Thomas' statement to the ACS, on May 26, 1975, the *New York Times* carried an article on an alleged West Coast ring to smuggle banned cancer drugs.[252] It told how an assistant US attorney was preparing Grand Jury indictments against top leaders of the laetrile movement, including Ernst T. Krebs, Jr., Andrew McNaughton and Ernesto Contreras. These were the same men who had been respectfully consulted by SKI not long before, but their involvement with laetrile was now being interpreted as "an international smuggling operation," comparable, said one government official, to "Mexican brown heroin traffic." This fruit kernel extract that was relied upon by thousands of "terminal" cancer patients was being compared to a deadly and illicit street drug!

Justification for the government's prosecution came from the statements of Memorial Sloan-Kettering's esteemed president at the ACS Science Writer's Seminar. This included the claim that laetrile has absolutely no value either in combating cancer, prolonging life or inhibiting tumor growth.

Absolutely no value! Sitting in my office, one floor below his own, I contemplated this statement over and over again, trying to find some way to justify or explain it. I could find none.

Thomas' statements may even have been timed to coordinate with the actions of the FDA and Justice Department to imprison, fine and otherwise incapacitate the leaders of the laetrile movement. In any case, I was now convinced that there was some sort of cover-up underway, and that Thomas was part of it.

If SKI denied that there ever had been positive results, how safe were the notes Sugiura had shown me the year before? What would happen if he died (he was 83)? I foresaw SKI disposing of all the positive laboratory notes and memos, and then issuing a totally fabricated negative report on its testing.

Thomas' April 2nd statement to the ACS prompted me to ask Sugiura if he would join me for lunch in Manhattan to help celebrate my 32nd birthday on May 6. When he said yes, I asked (as nonchalantly as I could) if he would bring along copies of his laetrile lab results. He asked me why, of course, and I explained—rather implausibly, I feared—that I needed them to round out a picture of his recent activities for an article on him for *Center News*. To my amazement, he agreed to bring me a copy.

My heart was in my mouth when, sitting down in a restaurant near the hospital, he handed me a thick interoffice envelope containing all the lab notes on his experiments. What amazing results these were! To my knowledge, nothing that he or anyone else at SKI had worked on had yielded results comparable to those with laetrile. Admittedly, laetrile did not shrink established tumors or extend the lifespan of the mice. But the profound effect on metastases was obvious in the treatment and prevention experiments.

I now had his notes in hand. I asked my mother-in-law to keep a copy in her safe deposit box in a Brooklyn bank. Perhaps I was being overly cautious, but I feared that the government might raid my apartment once they learned that Sugiura had given me copies. I then began to judiciously show photocopies to a few select individuals.

Because I was repelled by the politics of the John Birch Society and its front group, the Committee for Freedom of Choice in Cancer, Inc., I hoped to interest some liberal or left wing group in this topic. But, to my dismay, I ran into a wall of opposition on the left. I was turned down, sometimes rudely, by almost everyone I contacted. Many people I found had ties to academic medicine, and the "John Birch Society Connection"[253] had irredeemably tainted laetrile in the eyes of most liberals. If the John Birch Society, whose founder claimed that President Dwight D. Eisenhower was a Communist, was for it, they were against it. I simply didn't know where to turn.

The most likely "progressive" group at that time was Science for the People. Like me, many of its members had roots in the anti-Vietnam War movement of the 1960s. As some of their scientists moved up the ladder they had become a kind of radical caucus of the American Association for the Advancement of Science (AAAS).

I started to attend their meetings in Manhattan and to raise the laetrile issue. This led to strident arguments. People picked holes in the theory behind laetrile and especially in its connection to the extreme right wing. I still felt that, theory and politics aside, Sugiura's work spoke for itself. I eventually found a few like-minded individuals, especially one City University of New York (CUNY) biochemistry graduate student named Alec Pruchnicki. Alec (who later became a medical doctor in New York City) grasped the importance of Sugiura's scientific findings and how they were being suppressed. He became a close colleague and participant throughout the laetrile controversy.

Eventually, the New York chapter of Science for the People endorsed a statement that called on SKI to publish the record of its laetrile testing. But even this mild statement was enormously controversial within the group, especially with the dominant Boston chapter. My strong impression, from this and other encounters, was that the left as a whole was unreceptive to "complementary and alternative medicine." That only changed when the liberal Senator Tom Harkin (D-IA) promoted research into CAM at the NIH, starting in the 1990s.

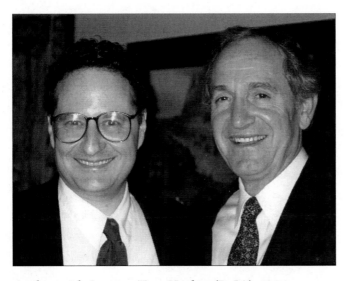

Author with Senator Tom Harkin (D-IA), 1994

Jane Brody Article

I also decided to show Sugiura's documents to someone in the media who might expose the whole situation. That summer I contacted Jane Brody, the celebrated medical writer of the *New York Times*. It was a gamble. I knew she had written *You Can Fight Cancer—and Win!* (1974) with the ACS's executive vice president Arthur Holleb, MD, but I didn't yet know about his fateful letter to Bob Good. To me, she seemed like a fair and influential reporter.

An exposé by her would certainly have set the record straight about Sugiura's experiments. She asked me to meet her in the *Times'* science newsroom, at the paper's old headquarters just off Times Square. We chatted for a while (she had been at Cornell University at the same time as my older brother) and I then handed her a photocopy of Sugiura's notes and explained their significance. She was friendly, but said that she never wanted to write about laetrile and went into the topic reluctantly.

Shortly after this, I was sitting in Jerry's office when she called and announced that she wanted an exclusive interview on laetrile with all the top leaders of the institution. Although they seemed to be friendly (Jerry revealed that they were in fact tennis partners), he explained that he had promised many people that he would release the results to all reporters simultaneously. She then said that she had seen a copy of Sugiura's lab notes, but would not say where she had gotten it.

She came to SKI and held interviews with top officials. I then waited. And waited. And waited, until I began to think nothing would come of it. I went on my summer vacation and as my wife and I were driving on the New York Thruway we stopped to pick up a paper. There, finally, was Brody's article, on page one.[254]

"Now the truth will finally come out," I told Martha, excitedly. But the article was exactly the opposite of what I expected and hoped for. In the article, Brody quoted officials saying that Sugiura's extensive results were "spurious" and the result of "the vagaries of experimental variation" and "unfamiliarity with the animals used." She was talking about a man who had caught experimental rats in the basement of Roosevelt Hospital before World War I! He had also used the Swiss albino mouse system, in which he also saw positive laetrile results, since World War II. He had worked with BALB/c mice[255] and their offshoot, CD8F1 mice, for years.[256]

Throughout this ordeal, Sugiura said nothing in public to contradict the misstatements of his superiors. He maintained the attitude that it was up to "downtown" to sort out what they would do with his results. His job was to conduct research, not get involved in controversy. But he repeatedly emphasized that in nearly 60 years no one had ever found cause to contradict his work. He also would refuse to put his name to the final paper unless his complete data were included.

Medical World News

The second reporter with whom I shared Sugiura's data was David N. Leff (1918-2004) of McGraw Hill's biweekly magazine, *Medical World News*. He seemed like a reasonably objective person. But having gotten through the *New York Times* interview unscathed, Stock now felt emboldened. In the course of his interview with Leff, he unequivocally stated:

> *"We have found amygdalin negative in all the animal systems we have tested."*[257]

Good and Thomas were "political scientists" as Gerry and I jokingly called them, but I thought that the dry-as-dust Stock would always remain technically accurate in his statements. But there was simply no way that this unambiguous statement could be squared with the truth. Reading this statement was a turning point in my appraisal of him. Up until then, I was inclined to give him the benefit of the doubt. But at this point I realized that Stock had become an integral part of an organized effort to denigrate Sugiura's results.

As a reminder, at the time that Stock made this statement to *Medical World News* (August 1975) there had already been:

- Positive results in 6 treatment experiments in CD8F1 mice (Sugiura)

- Positive results in 1 prevention experiment in CD8F1 mice (Sugiura)

- Somewhat positive results in AKR leukemia mice (Sugiura)

- Positive results in Swiss Albino mice (Sugiura and Jacobs-Schloen)

- Positive results in the first Stockert experiment (although never acknowledged as such).

So, to say that SKI had found laetrile "negative in all the animal systems tested" was the absolute opposite of the truth. Jumping ahead, in November 1977, after I helped bring the mendacity of this quotation to the attention of the public, Stock wrung his hands in despair. He claimed that he had been misquoted by the *Medical World News* reporter, David Leff. In a memo to MSKCC employees, Stock wrote in reference to this statement:

"I'll never live down the misquote I should have corrected."[258]

At least he realized that he would never live down this statement. But claiming that this was a "misquote" put the onus on the person who did the quoting, in this case David Leff, and not on the person giving him the quote, namely himself. Stock didn't have the good graces to say that he had "misspoken," but rather that the reporter had "misquoted" him. When I later told Leff about Stock's response, he just smiled and quietly reaffirmed that he had quoted him correctly. I believed him because reporters of his experience did not often misquote their sources.

But even in the unlikely event that Leff had indeed misquoted him, Stock had had two years to correct this error. That is what a person would normally do if a false statement of great importance were attributed to him.

Obviously, this was no random "misquote." Stock's comments were in sync with Good's statement of January 10, 1974 and Thomas' of May 1975. Stock had simply fallen into line with his own superiors. But mulling over this *Medical World News* article, I realized that Sloan-Kettering had hardened its stance: put another way, the fix was in.

Why would Stock do this? In my opinion, he was the Organization Man[259] par excellence, who subordinated his personal desires to the demands of his institution. Stock wasn't lying about laetrile on his own account or out of malice, He was doing it for the greater good of the Organization, as he perceived it.

But at that moment, sitting in my office with a fresh copy of *Medical World News* in front of me, I thought: "You work for liars and you yourself are in danger of becoming their accomplice." I felt alternate surges of anger and despair.

Clinical trials? "No way!"

One of the big questions before the "establishment" was whether or not to do a human clinical trial with laetrile. It may surprise some readers that in the years in question, it was the FDA, not the laetrilists, who stood in the way of performing such a clinical trial. As I have said, the McNaughton Foundation (which supplied the laetrile for Sloan-Kettering's experiments) had long sought to sponsor such a trial in human patients. It had even obtained an Investigative New Drug (IND) number for laetrile in 1970, only to have that permit yanked from it by the FDA eight days later.[260]

In March 1974 the FDA Commissioner, Alexander M. Schmidt, warned researchers not to attempt to perform clinical trials with laetrile, or to face criminal charges. He was quoted as follows:

> "If someone does proceed with clinical trials [with laetrile,
> ed.] he will be in violation of the law and we will take
> action."[261]

In other words, laetrile doesn't work…and don't you dare try to prove that it does!

In 1975 Old had invited the Mexico City oncologist, Mario Soto de Leon, MD, as a guest on "13 Howard," as he actively tried to arrange a collaborative trial of laetrile at the 20th of November Hospital. Earlier that year Old had written to Soto on SKI stationery:

> "It was indeed a pleasure to have you and Dr. Sannen visit
> our Institute and share with us your clinical experience with
> amygdalin in cancer patients. I was pleased to hear from Dr.
> Sannen that our proposed collaborative controlled trials
> have the approval of your hospital. We are looking forward
> to a fruitful exchange of information."[262]

This was the clinical trial that was agreed upon at the NCI conclave. Yet, less than a year later, in a complete about face, SKI officials vehemently denied that there was any scientific reason to perform a clinical trial.

Benno Schmidt, who as Cancer Czar had initiated the laetrile experiments, told *Medical World News* on the topic of clinical trials:

> *"No way. There's no way, I believe, that they can convince the people at Sloan-Kettering there's any basis for going further."*

I realized that an exposé of Sugiura's testing would not emerge through a blockbuster article in the *New York Times* or probably any other national publication. My overtures to left-wing publications had proved futile. My brief involvement with Science for the People had come to naught. I was truly at an impasse.

Realizing that Sugiura's results had been twisted into unrecognizable shape, I put a sheet of MSKCC stationery in my typewriter and addressed an anonymous letter to Michael Culbert of the Committee for Freedom of Choice in Cancer, Inc. This was a step that I had been trying to avoid when I gave a copy of the notes to Jane Brody. I walked to the corner of First Avenue and 68th Street and, taking a deep breath, dropped a large packet of information into the mailbox.

Within a week the Committee for Freedom of Choice announced receipt of Sugiura's lab notes. Under the title *Anatomy of a Cover-Up*, with a commentary by Ernst T. Krebs, Jr. (co-inventor of laetrile) they began selling copies of these to people around the world.

Sugiura's results, once their impact registered at "Freedom of Choice" headquarters in Los Altos, Calif., received considerable attention in "alternative medicine" circles. But it had little impact on the general population. It was seen as just more pro-laetrile propaganda, and as a consequence was regarded as inherently unreliable. The leak of this information proved to be only a speed bump for the SKI administration, once they had joined the ACS and NCI in their campaign to negate Sugiura's findings.

"Blind" Study Announced

One temporary victory was that in November 1975, Stock announced a new "blind" study of laetrile.[263] Jerry Delaney told the Associated Press:

> *"The researchers who conduct the study will not know which mice are being given laetrile, and which mice a dummy substance."*[264]

But Sloan-Kettering leaders, who a short while before had pleaded with the FDA and NCI to allow them to participate in the Mexican clinical trial, now told the AP:

> *"There does not appear to be sufficient scientific data to justify clinical trials, that is, trials with human patients, with the controversial drug."*

"No way!" Benno Schmidt exclaimed.

What had changed was not the science, but the politics. To be blunt, the NCI had finally had placed its own man within the Sloan-Kettering program. This was Daniel Martin, who was creating havoc, confusion and demoralization in the SKI ranks. Old, with his shy personality, was simply no match for someone who could declare, in the face of Sugiura's meticulous data that laetrile was without activity in spontaneous tumors in mice—period.[265]

The Stockert Challenge

Stockert's first and second experiments are discussed on page 92 of the final SKI laetrile paper with data given in Table VII on page 101. The Jacobs-Schloen experiment is discussed in the Second Opinion Special Report *and in* Medical World News.

I now will deal with the four major challenges that SKI used in an attempt to contradict Sugiura's results. These came from three scientists at SKI itself (Stockert, Schmid and Stock) and one from Catholic Medical Center (Martin). Documentary evidence for their studies is derived from the SKI Paper itself.

Elisabeth S. Stockert, DPhil, was born in Austria on September 29, 1930. She came from one of the richest families in Europe. Her maternal great grandfather was Karl Wittgenstein (1847-1913), who controlled an effective monopoly on iron and steel resources in the pre-WWI Austro-Hungarian Empire. Her grandmother was Karl's daughter, Helene "Lenka" Wittgenstein Salzer (1879-1956), who was the sister of the celebrated Anglo-Austrian philosopher Ludwig Wittgenstein (1889-1951).

Stockert came to the US in 1959 to work on chemotherapy at SKI, but after "Dusty" Rhoads' sudden death from a heart attack that year she transferred to Lloyd Old's immunology group.[266] She then worked closely with Old as a member of his inner circle, until her own death from cancer in September 2002.

Almost all of her 139 publications were coauthored with Old, and she was first author of only eight of these. According to a colleague, she was "a close personal friend of Lloyd and a major contributor to Lloyd's research legacy."[267]

SKI first asked Stockert to reproduce Sugiura's work. She claimed that her experiments refuted Sugiura's conclusions, but, closely examined, such claims were distorted and one-sided. Stockert never provided adequate details on her two solo experiments with laetrile. Her one public accounting, in *Medical World News* in October 1975, was garbled. She conflated the two experiments that she had performed and omitted any mention of an unpublished positive experiment that had been performed in her lab (and which only came to light two years later).

Yet Stock repeatedly used Stockert's work to contradict Sugiura's findings. For instance, the SKI paper states:

> "*Consequent experiments independently by Stockert…also failed to confirm Sugiura's initial observations.*"

This claim, however, requires further commentary.

Stockert's First Experiment

In a description of her first experiment in the final paper Stockert says:

> "*Experimental conditions were the same as in Dr. Sugiura's experiments except that in the first of the 2 experiments the mice received a different diet*" (p. 92).

However, this was not completely true. In her first laetrile experiment, Stockert used a dose of 1,000/mg/kg/day of laetrile, which was half of what Sugiura normally used. She never explained why she used a dose of 1,000 mg/kg/day or why (by saying that she had merely changed the diet) she implied that she had used the same dose as Sugiura.

Stockert claimed that she was unable to reproduce Sugiura's positive findings in lung metastases, and expressed regret over this. But the data that she provided in the SKI paper (p. 99) suggested a much more nuanced picture. Macrovisually, which was the only way she examined the mice, she reported metastases in 7 out of 13 (or 54 percent) of the control mice vs. 3 out of 10 (or 30 percent) of the laetrile-treated mice. In what way though was this negative for laetrile? Even at a half dose, there was an absolute reduction of 24 percent metastases in the laetrile-treated mice. According to my statistical consultant, the relative risk (RR) of metastases was 0.557 in this experiment. But because the sample size was too small to draw statistical conclusions from the results, technically speaking there was no statistically significant difference in the probability of metastases between the two groups.

But to me, the trend was clear. In Sugiura's first experiment (the only one in which he also used a half-dose) he found an identical percentage of laetrile-treated mice with lung metastases, i.e., 30 percent. But since he saw metastases in 8 out of 10 control animals, the difference between the two was a 66.3 percent reduction, which, according to my statistician, was highly significant.

There was one logical explanation for there being fewer lung metastases in the control animals. This occurred when a researcher sacrificed the control animals prematurely. Their cancers simply didn't have sufficient time to develop to the point of becoming visually detectable. This in turn rendered laetrile's advantage statistically insignificant.

We know that CD8F1 mice, when allowed to die of their disease developed lung metastases in a higher percent of cases than Stockert reported. For example, in August 1974, Martin reported that 73 percent of untreated CD8F1 mice normally developed lung metastases in the course of their lifetime.[268] Sugiura usually found lung metastases in around 80 percent of the saline-injected control mice and MSKCC pathologists typically found a similar, albeit somewhat smaller, percentage. But anyone reporting a much lower percentage of metastases in the control animals was almost certainly sacrificing the animals prematurely, before they had a chance to develop their full complement of metastases.

Stockert told *Medical World News* that in her first experiment she did not allow the control mice to die a natural death, but sacrificed them when "they looked very sick and were not likely to live any longer."[269] But this was a subjective determination and in her case seems to have been premature. Had she allowed the control mice to live out their natural lifespan, more metastases would probably have developed, which would have then brought her results into closer alignment with those of Sugiura.

Although the data in her first experiment trended in laetrile's advantage this was interpreted as a refutation, not a confirmation, of Sugiura's results.

This was part and parcel of the falsehood that no one at Sloan-Kettering was ever able to confirm Sugiura's experimental results.

Stockert's Second Experiment

In her second experiment, Stockert let the animals live longer and then reported 67 percent metastases in the controls. But this time, instead of 30 percent metastases in the laetrile-treated animals, she reported 65 percent.

In her October 11, 1975 *Medical World News* interview, Stockert claimed to see no difference between the two groups:

> *"I found that I didn't see any difference between the amygdalin and the control mice, and I was rather upset by it. Actually, the laetrile mice looked sicker to me than the control mice, so I sacrificed them much earlier."*[270]

This once again brings up the question of how one properly determines the presence of lung metastases in experimental animals. In both of her tests Stockert used only the macrovisual method of determining metastases and failed to submit the animals' lungs to the MSKCC Pathology Department for independent verification (as Sugiura did). In her interview with David Leff of *Medical World News* she gave a half-hearted explanation for why she failed to do so:

> *"She also checked her subjective macroscopic impressions against those of a pathologist in her office, who agreed with her. They decided against a histologic [microscopic, ed.] examination because visible results were so clear-cut."*[271]

But in the SKI Paper, three years later, Stockert failed to mention this pathologist. Who was this mysterious person who visually confirmed the presence of metastases in the mice? No name is given. He or she might have been an SKI employee employed in her laboratory or perhaps just a visitor passing through. In either case, the question is moot since a pathologist qua pathologist is a person who utilizes a microscope to examine suspect tissue. But this office pathologist only used his or her eyeballs and decided against performing a microscopic examination. So, at best, this was a third party's macrovisual impression. It was far from a scientific determination, such as was made by the five MSKCC pathologists who routinely used their microscopes to double-check the results in Sugiura's experiments.

It was almost comical how SKI leaders tried to have it both ways. They readily accepted Stockert's macrovisual method of detecting metastases when this seemingly undermined the credibiliy of Sugiura's results. But they also subjected this same method to withering criticism when they erroneously claimed that this was how Sugiura had detected fewer metastases in laetrile-treated mice.

Of course, it cannot be stated often enough that the SKI paper is totally wrong when it attributes these "subjective determinations" to Sugiura, to whom they did not apply. The criticism in fact emphatically applied to Stockert.

The Jacobs-Schloen Experiment

Stockert's credibility was further undermined by the fact that she failed to mention a positive laetrile experiment performed in her own laboratory. This was the so-called Jacobs-Schloen experiment in Swiss Albino mice. Ms. Shelly Jacobs was an SKI technician; Lloyd H. Schloen, PhD was an SKI Postdoctoral Fellow, working under Lloyd Old. The reader will recall that he was one of the two individuals whom Old sent to Baden-Baden in 1973 as SKI's spokesperson. Together, Jacobs and Schloen (under Old's overall direction) undertook an experiment with laetrile in Swiss Albino mice.

The experiment began in the fall of 1973. It proceeded without incident until December 1973, when Stockert left on a visit to Paris. In her absence, Jacobs and Schloen simply completed the experiment, which Jacobs then summarized in a January 1974 memorandum to Old. This summation was highly positive in nature.

I learned about the existence of this experiment completely by accident in early 1976. Upon completing his 1973-1975 fellowship, Schloen came to work in the Development department that adjoined Public Affairs on the 20th floor. Lloyd Schloen and I soon became friends. We shared an interest in unconventional treatments and he casually mentioned to me some laetrile experiments with Swiss Albino mice of which I was then unaware.

Jacobs had left the institution, but Schloen managed to recover a copy of her memo to Old. In this memo, Jacobs was brimming with barely concealed excitement: the Swiss Albino mice receiving the highest dose of laetrile appeared healthy at the time of sacrifice, whereas those receiving lower doses, or saline solution, were very sick, the exact opposite of what Stockert claimed to observe in her second experiment.

When this eventually came to light, Stockert replied that because the experiment had been completed while she was in Paris, she did not trust the results and was therefore justified in omitting them from any further discussion.

There does not appear to be anything wrong with this experiment, however, and it should have been included in the plus column in any consideration of laetrile's effects. Instead, it was suppressed.

The Schmid Challenge

Schmid's first and second experiments are discussed on page 100 of the final SKI laetrile paper with tabulated data in Table VIII on page 101.

The second major challenge to Sugiura's results came from the Walker Laboratory chemotherapy researcher, Franz A. Schmid, DVM, who was involved in a total of three laetrile experiments (SKI paper, pp. 100-104). What made his participation fraught with difficulty was that he was Sugiura's son-in-law, married to Kanematsu's only child, his daughter Miyono. Together with Sugiura's Belgian-born wife, Zoe Marie, they all lived together in Harrison, NY. In fact, Kanematsu, Franz and Miyono had published a scientific paper together in 1961.[272]

Stock, with scores of Walker Lab scientists to choose from, had assigned Franz Schmid of all people the task of replicating his father-in-law's work. A refutation of Sugiura's findings by Schmid would be devastating, as critics could then declare, "See, his own son-in-law could not confirm his work!" But a confirmation could be greeted with "Well, what did you expect, it's his son-in-law!" It was a classic no-win situation.

In the SKI laetrile paper, Schmid's presentation of his three experiments lacks the detail seen in Sugiura's contribution. But, as we shall see, in the end Schmid's work did not refute Sugiura's findings but confirmed them!

Schmid's First Experiment

In Schmid's first experiment there were 20 laetrile-treated animals and 19 controls. Treated animals received Sugiura's standard dose of 2,000 mg/kg/day of laetrile, while control animals received injections of inert saline solution. The average survival time of the treated animals was 53 days vs. 40 days for the controls. This represented a 13-day absolute increase for laetrile. These apparently positive effects went un-remarked in the SKI paper. My statistician pointed out that the raw survival times for animals in the Schmid experiments are not given in the SKI laetrile paper and he cannot determine if this increase in survival is statistically significant.

Schmid's Second Experiment

In Schmid's second experiment, there were 10 CD8F1 mice that received laetrile vs. 9 saline control animals. The astonishing thing about this experiment was that the dose of laetrile given was slashed to a mere 40 mg/kg/day, which was one-fiftieth of what Sugiura used in his experiments. Despite this, the average survival of laetrile-treated animals was 63 days vs. 41 days in the controls. This represents an absolute increase of 21 days. But the SKI paper states the following:

> "*In neither of the 2 [Schmid, ed.] experiments was there a significant difference in...survival time...between the control and treated groups*" (p. 94).

The key word here is "significant." SKI is saying that the results were not statistically significant. In other words we cannot rule out the possibility that they were due to chance. Again, my statistics consultant commented that "the significance in survival times between the two groups could not be calculated due to the lack of raw data in the paper."

That said, the trend of the data seems clear. Mice in the laetrile-treated group lived longer, although the experiment was too small to definitively attribute this to a treatment effect.

I might note that Schmid's second experiment almost brought an abrupt end to my career at MSKCC. The tiny dose of laetrile caused no positive effect on lung metastases when judged macrovisually, although laetrile-treated mice lived longer. Nevertheless, Stock seized on this experiment as a tie-breaking failure for laetrile.

Jerry Delaney passed along instructions for me to drop everything and write a press release on the "failure of laetrile" in the second Schmid experiment. On Stock's instructions, we would then release this story to the numerous reporters to whom we had promised a closing story on the testing of this controversial agent.

Initially, I accepted Schmid's study as a failure to confirm his father-in-law's work. But, as part of my own due diligence, I phoned Sugiura to ask for a comment. I thought he might concede defeat but after hesitating for a moment he said, tersely, "Ask Dr. Schmid what dose he used in his experiment."

I had assumed without question (as most people would) that the dose would be the typical 2,000 mg/kg/day. This was not only Sugiura's dose but the same as Schmid himself had used in his first experiment. How could it be anything else, since a confirmatory study implied replication of all of the previous test conditions? Later that afternoon, I reached Schmid at his laboratory and introduced myself as a fellow MSKCC employee.

"I am writing up the latest laetrile experiment, and I'd like to ask you a question," I said.

He immediately sounded suspicious. "Where are you from?" he demanded, in his brusque German accent.

"I'm from here," I stammered. "Memorial Sloan-Kettering. Our Department of Public Affairs."

"What is the question?"

"What was the dose of laetrile you used in your latest experiment."

Without further comment, he hung up the phone! Astonished, I called back, repeatedly, but now got only a busy signal.

Amazed at this bizarre behavior, which was unprecedented for me at SKI, I called Stock and, as calmly as I could, said, "I am in the process of writing up Dr. Schmid's laetrile experiment as you requested."

"Good, good," he said, sounding pleased.

"But I do have one question that I need to have answered."

"Ask away." For a dour man he seemed almost ebullient, as if he finally saw an end to his laetrile troubles.

My voice was a little shaky, but I pushed on.

"What was the dose that Dr. Schmid used in his experiment?"

"The dose?" Stock hesitated for a moment and then said, "Forty milligrams per kilogram." One didn't need to know higher math to realize that this was a small fraction of what Sugiura had routinely used.

Suddenly I realized I was on thin ice. I was after all talking to a vice president of Sloan-Kettering Institute and I didn't want to pursue the question in a way that openly challenged his authority, much less his honesty. Still, the question demanded answering.

"But, Dr. Stock" I said, "In his experiments Dr. Sugiura used 2,000 milligrams per kilogram." I hesitated. "Are you saying that Dr. Schmid used only one-fiftieth of that dose?"

"That's right," Stock said, starting to sound a little testy.

"But why?" I stammered.

"I authorized that dose," said Stock, "because it was more comparable to the three grams per day being taken orally by some patients."

This was delivered with such effortlessness that it sounded as though it had been rehearsed. Stock was telling me he had cut Sugiura's dose fiftyfold, and now wanted me to announce this without comment as a failure to replicate his earlier results.

Struggling to keep my composure I said: "Dr. Stock, Dr. Schmid's results may be negative, but I don't think one can say that he has reproduced Dr. Sugiura's experiment in any meaningful sense."

"I wouldn't be too concerned about that," Stock said, coldly. "Just write up the results and say that Dr. Schmid has found laetrile negative in his latest experiment."

"I'll work on it," I said vaguely, and hung up.

I spent the weekend mulling over this proposition and discussing it with my family. If I hadn't called Sugiura, and if he hadn't advised me to call Schmid, I might never have learned about this glaring discrepancy in the doses. I felt that if I wrote the press release the way Stock wanted, I would be sucked into the quicksand of a widening cover-up. That was not why I had signed up for my otherwise excellent job.

Obviously, the smart thing to do would be to just write the press release. This would have earned me some kudos from my boss, maybe even helped me get a raise on my next anniversary. It would also have doomed Sugiura's work to oblivion.

My need to hold onto my job was great. I had two small children at home and, like most young couples, Martha and I struggled to pay our bills each month. I hadn't yet learned what the sociologist Robert Jackall has mordantly called "the fundamental rules" of corporate life:

*"Your job is not to report something that your boss does not
want reported, but rather to cover it up. You do your job and
you keep your mouth shut."*[273]

Every Monday morning at 9 am the professional members of the Public
Affairs Department held a meeting to discuss the work of the coming
week. These were usually pleasant and relaxed occasions among seven or
eight friendly colleagues.

That Monday, I explained to my colleagues what had happened in
Schmid's experiment. I could see Jerry's face transition through all the
flesh tones between pale pink and cherry red. I knew that he agreed with
me on many of the contradictions in SKI's position on laetrile and part of
him was skeptical of authority, as many people were in that post-Water-
gate era. But he was nervous over how far I intended to take my revolt.
Finally, I said:

*"I don't think I can write that Schmid's experiment was
negative, without also pointing out that he used one-fiftieth
of Sugiura's normal dose."*

Jerry had done me many good turns, starting with the fact that he had
hired me when that idea seemed a bit far-fetched. He had given me the
start of a wonderful new career. He also had encouraged me to investigate
Sugiura's work. I got raises every year and eventually he even made me
Assistant Director of the Department. Generally speaking, he was a good
boss, and more than fair to me personally.

But now he was upset and even agitated.

"You can put that in a memo to Dr. Stock," he said, tersely, "but I'd
better warn you that you'll probably be fired for insubordination."

The other staff members went silent; they seemed confused and embarrassed. For most of them, this was the first they had heard about the
Schmid experiment.

"So be it," I said. I abruptly got up from my chair and went back to my
office. I quickly called Martha and told her what was happening, then put
a sheet of stationery with a carbon copy into my IBM Selectric and started

typing up my refusal. I knew that sending the letter would probably result in my termination. But I was in a grimly determined mood.

Before I could finish the letter, however, Jerry came tearing into my office. "Don't send that memo," he said, excitedly. "I'll talk to Dr. Stock." What had changed his mind? After I left the meeting, my fellow professional staff members had informed Jerry that they would co-sign my letter. One "disgruntled employee" could be explained away, but hardly a rebellion of the entire professional staff, which might have cost Jerry his own job. So he wisely reversed himself and agreed to negotiate the issue with Stock.

The upshot was that I never had to write the Schmid press release, nor did anyone else. Instead, the SKI administration decided to conduct yet another experiment. This was to be a final "tie-breaker" in which Schmid and Sugiura would collaborate by observing the same animals. This was a small, albeit temporary, victory. After my conversation with Stock, however, I realized that he would stretch the truth to achieve the result that he desired. I may have slowed the juggernaut, but I had hardly stopped it.

Schmid-Sugiura Collaboration

The Schmid-Sugiura Collaboration is discussed on page 100 of the final SKI laetrile paper with tabulated data in Table VIII on page 101.

In late 1975, Schmid and Sugiura began their collaborative experiment at the Walker Lab. CD8F1 mice were treated until they died natural deaths (which allowed for the maximum number of metastases to develop in each group). The two scientists then made independent macrovisual evaluations of the animals' lungs. But this time, unlike in Schmid's (or Stockert's) other experiments, macrovisual observations were followed by microscopic examinations of lung tissue by the MSKCC pathologists assigned to this project.

The results came out significantly in laetrile's favor (see SKI paper p. 100 and 104).

Specifically, Schmid found by macrovisual observation that there were 80 percent lung metastases in the controls vs. 44 percent in the laetrile-treated mice. There was thus a 36 percent absolute decrease in lung metastases. This was, as the SKI paper itself states, statistically significant with a p value of 0.04, meaning there was only a 1-in-25 chance that these results were achieved by happenstance.

My statistical consultant, Prof. Mahoney, recalculated the raw data given in the paper and came up with a p value of 0.0246 (even better than was stated in the SKI paper). The relative risk of metastasis was calculated as 0.547, meaning that there was about one-half the chance of developing metastases in the laetrile group.

Sugiura detected metastases in 100 percent of the control animals vs. 38 percent in the treated mice. This represented a 62 percent decrease in metastases in the laetrile-treated mice. Mahoney, using the Chi-square test, saw a statistically significant difference in the probability of metastases between the laetrile-treated and the control groups. (In this case the relative risk was 0.375).

At the same time, the MSKCC pathology department, using microscopic analysis, detected 80 percent metastases in the controls vs. just 31 percent in the laetrile-treated animals. This represented an absolute decrease of 49 percent in lung metastases in the laetrile-treated mice. The relative decrease observed by the pathologists was similar to that seen by both Schmid and Sugiura.

Prof. Mahoney's overall conclusion was as follows:

> *"By the measurements of all three observers, there was a significant difference in the probability of any metastases between the two cohorts."*

Thus, all observers unequivocally confirmed the fact that laetrile inhibited metastases in the lungs of CD8F1 mice.

This confirmation could have provided a fitting end to the entire SKI laetrile experiment. Yet, Stock would not allow these results to be published at the time. As he later told Nicholas Wade of *Science*:

> *"If we had published those early positive data, it would have caused all kind of havoc."*[274]

Years later, when it came time for publication, the 1978 SKI paper never even commented on the positive outcome of the Schmid-Sugiura Collaborative Experiment. Here is how the SKI paper described the three Schmid experiments, including his confirmatory Collaborative Experiment with Sugiura:

> *"There is concordance in the results of the first 2 experiments with respect to percentage of mice with lung metastases, even though the dosages given were quite different. For the same criteria the first and third experiments at the same dosage present opposing results; however, in the third experiment there is some discrepancy between individuals (F.S. and K.S.) in evaluation of the number of mice with lung metastases."*

This is a classic instance of scientific gobbledygook. Most readers could never discover from this convoluted passage that both observers (Schmid and Sugiura) saw significantly positive effects of laetrile on lung metastases. Nor was there any acknowledgement that the MSKCC Pathology Department had confirmed both scientists' visual observations by use of standard microscopic techniques. In other words, laetrile worked significantly well in this experiment, but SKI did everything in its power to obscure that fact.

As I wrote in 1977:

> *"Anyone who can figure out from this explanation that Schmid had in fact confirmed Sugiura's findings is remarkably perceptive."*[275]

To add insult to injury, at the SKI Press Conference, Stock outrageously tried to pass off the Schmid-Sugiura Collaborative Test as a failure for laetrile. Here is what he wrote in the version of the SKI laetrile paper that was released at the press conference of June 15, 1977:

"All experiments of 3 independent observers [Stockert,
Schmid and Martin, ed.]...have failed to confirm Sugiura's
initial results."[276]

That's right, all of the experiments of Schmid, which would necessarily include the collaborative test with Sugiura, were negative! One astute reporter at the press conference asked Schmid about this discrepancy. He grudgingly acknowledged the confirmatory study, before becoming nonplussed and handing the microphone to Dr. Good. Here is how the dialog went:

Reporter: "In fact, in your third test, did you in effect confirm Dr. Sugiura's findings?"

Schmid: "Yeah, in the third test, yes. But that is two to one."

Reporter: "And in the second test, you used a very small dosage of amygdalin."

Schmid: "Yeah, that's true."

Reporter: "Okay, then why don't you state in the findings that one of your independent investigators confirmed Dr. Sugiura?"

Good (taking the microphone from Schmid): "If you read the paper, we do bring forth every bit of evidence and we discuss it."

In the published version of the paper, (because of *Second Opinion's* exposé) SKI emended this sentence to read:

"An additional experiment by Schmid and Sugiura gave
results in the same direction as Sugiura's early observations,
significant with a p value of 0.04 in Schmid's evaluation,
while that by Sugiura was more highly significant" (p. 121).

Only in "the same direction"? Both observations were positive and statistically significant. What did it matter that Sugiura's results were slightly more positive than Schmid's? They were both positive. Schmid confirmed Sugiura's observations, as had the MSKCC pathology department.

But this was as close as SKI ever came to admitting that the Collaborative Test had actually confirmed the efficacy of laetrile. The confirmation by pathologists was not commented on (much less accounted for) in the final SKI paper. Instead, they lied in saying that Sugiura's results were based on his macrovisual observations—a naked, bald and easily refuted lie, had enough people bothered to read the 34-page paper. But, as Stock laughingly said at the press conference, few people bother to read scientific papers. Even many scientists content themselves with a paper's Abstract, which as a rule only contains the main authors' conclusions, not raw data that might contradict those conclusions.

Instead of embracing Schmid's confirmatory results, and publishing the paper that Sugiura sent to him in January 1976, Stock called for yet another experiment. Sugiura just couldn't win this battle: no matter how many times he repeated his positive results, even after another scientist confirmed them, SKI continued to seek a negative answer.

Emboldened by his million-dollar grant from the NCI, and his newfound position as chief 'quackbuster' of the American Society of Clinical Oncology, Martin ramped up his crusade to destroy the laetrile movement. He would not be deterred by anything as simple as a positive laboratory test by Sugiura and Schmid.

Nicholas Wade of *Science*, summarizing Schmid's experiments, said:

> *"Another Sloan-Kettering researcher, Franz Schmid, conducted a trio of experiments with laetrile, in two of which the substance offered no sign of efficacy. In the third, however, laetrile showed a positive anti-tumor effect which was significant at the 0.04 level of probability.*
>
> *"The charge [of deception, ed.] has some merit, particularly when considered in the light of a key sentence in the summary of the report: 'All experiments of 3 independent observers...have failed to confirm Sugiura's initial results."*[277]

After the exposé in *Science* and elsewhere, Stock changed the relevant statement in the final paper to read:

> *"All independently conducted experiments of 3 independent observers ... have failed to confirm Sugiura's initial results."*[278]

It might take a few readings to grasp the subtle difference. By adding the words "independently conducted" to the word "experiments" Stock could thereby omit from consideration the positive collaborative experiment that Sugiura and Schmid had performed together.

But there was no way around it. This so-called tiebreaker study had unequivocally confirmed that laetrile greatly diminished the occurrence of metastases in CD8F1 mice.

The Martin Challenge

The Martin-Sugiura "First Collaborative Experiment" is discussed on page 105 of the SKI Paper. The Catholic Medical Center solo experiment is discussed on pages 105 and 112. The "Second Cooperative Experiment" is on page 112 and 113. The "First 'Blind' Test of Amygdalin" is discussed on pages 113. The tabulated data for all of these experiments is given on pages 106-109.

Starting in 1973, Daniel S. Martin, MD became one of the most outspoken opponents of laetrile in the US. He was never shy about voicing his opinions and one of these was that laetrile was absolutely devoid of any activity, and was in fact a conscious fraud. It not only didn't work, but it could not work. His categorically negative statements were founded on intense hostility towards "quackery" that predated his involvement with laetrile. His credibility rested on his impressive title and the fact that he had developed the mouse model that Sugiura had used in most of his experiments.

Martin claimed to have performed "hundreds if not thousands" of experiments with CD8F1 mice since its development in the late 1950s.[279] In the final SKI paper he describes his experience with this mouse as "extensive and unique" (p. 33). But there emerged many signs of sloppiness and incompetence in the way he carried out his experiments. His does not appear to have been a well managed laboratory.

Leaving aside for a moment Martin's obvious prejudice against the "fraud" of laetrile, we need to seriously consider his four experiments with this substance. For someone who claimed absolute mastery of the materials, these were marked by a surprising degree of incompetence, by laboratory irregularities and by an idiosyncratic method of detecting metastases. The incompetence may have been due to the dilemma in which he found himself at Catholic Medical Center, where his own laboratory had been relegated to an abandoned graffiti-covered TB hospital known as a "Siberia." He also suffered staffing problems, especially during the summer vacation season.

Martin's entry into laetrile testing began in 1973 with an attempt to collaborate with Sugiura on a laetrile experiment. The SKI paper calls this the First Collaborative Experiment. Although this was later interpreted as a failure for laetrile, that too was incorrect. The experiment was terminated due to sloppy injection procedures, as well as the inexplicable loss of test materials.

First Collaborative Experiment

After word of Sugiura's positive experiments got out, Sloan-Kettering agreed to do a joint experiment with Dr. Martin. At the time there was no awareness that Martin was hostile to laetrile. He was friendly towards immunology, and Old thought he might prove an ally in the program to test laetrile. This turned out to be a serious miscalculation.

This First Collaborative Experiment (SKI paper, p. 105) began on July 23, 1973. Sugiura, and a Walker Lab colleague, George S. Tarnowski, MD, traveled every week from Rye to Woodhaven, Queens, to participate in their joint experiment.

Problems surfaced immediately. Stock had requested 220 mice for this experiment. According to the original plan, half of each group would be 'sacrificed' after 42 days, while the other half would be allowed to live until they reached 90 days.[280] But on July 24, 1973, Ruth Fugmann, Martin's long-time coworker, told Stock that she had initiated their laetrile experiment the previous morning (in Sugiura's absence) and that only a total of 93 animals would be released for the experiment:

> *"For the present, we will have to limit the experimentation*
> *with amygdalin [laetrile, ed.] to this number, in that tumor-*
> *bearing animals must be used to satisfy other immediate*
> *obligations, and our available personnel is limited in this*
> *vacation season."[281]*

Then, instead of sacrificing the two groups of animals at six weeks and 90 days (12+ weeks), the animals would be sacrificed after the remarkably short periods of three-and-a-half weeks and five-and-a-half weeks, respectively. Since most of the animals at that point would only have developed very small tumors, and far fewer metastases, this was too early for any significant differences to appear between treated and untreated mice. Such a schedule would inevitably make laetrile seem less effective, since both groups would have low rates of metastases.

But according to figures given in the SKI paper (p. 112) inexplicably only 63 animals (not the previously specified 93) were available for evaluation. This "loss" of 30 animals went unremarked in the SKI paper. But what happened to these 30 missing mice? Perehaps they never entered the experiment at all. Another explanation, judging from Martin's other experiments, was that they died unexpectedly in the course of the experiment and their bodies had decomposed before the staff got around to checking the cages. This alone would have made the final results highly unreliable.

In the surviving group that was 'sacrificed' after three-and-a-half weeks, there were 4 out of 19 of control animals with metastases (21 percent) vs. 8 out of 19 in the laetrile treated animals (42 percent).

In the group sacrificed after five-and-a-half weeks there were 5 out of 21 animals with lung metastases in the controls (23 percent) vs. 4 out of 11 in the laetrile-treated group (36 percent). At first sight, this would seem detrimental to laetrile. But in neither case did the rate of metastases in the control animals come close to the 75 to 80 percent lung metastasis rate that occurred in CD8F1 mice in other experiments, including Martin's own.[282] Thus, the animals were being sacrificed too early to yield meaningful results, perhaps to accommodate the vacation schedules of Martin's staff.

The collaborative test was marked by the following problem:

- The unexplained absence of 30 mice from final consideration in the experiment.

- A much too short testing period.

- A macrovisual method of determining metastases, the very method that is emphatically rejected elsewhere in the SKI paper.

The authors of the SKI paper state:

> *"The small percentage of control mice with metastases…*
> *suggested that…the experiment had been terminated too*
> *early"* (p. 105).

A "too early" terminated experiment is an invalid experiment. Yet, despite this, Martin in his public statements, such as at the March 1975 NCI Conclave, the August 1975 *Medical World News* interview,[283] the June 1977 SKI press conference and the final SKI 1978 paper, insisted on calling this experiment a failure for laetrile. Thus, the paper states:

> *"No significant difference was observed between the control*
> *and treated groups with respect to percentage with lung*
> *metastases"* (p. 105).

Yet the authors had already told us that the experiment was terminated too early to detect any meaningful difference!

To reiterate, this test was declared invalid at the time of its performance and thus failed to draw any meaningful conclusions about the effect of laetrile in CD8F1 mice. Thirty mice had gone astray, and the remaining mice had been sacrificed too early, which was a sure-fire way of keeping the percentage of metastases between the two groups statistically insignificant. Yet, strangely, this failure of an experiment was "resurrected" as a negative test for laetrile in the SKI paper.

Martin's Independent Experiment

The "Catholic Medical Center Experiment with Amygdalin Against Spontaneous Mammary Tumors in CD8F1 Mice of Daniel S. Martin and Ruth A. Fugmann" is discussed on page 105 and 112 of the SKI Paper.

In July 1974, Martin carried out his own independent experiment with laetrile in CD8F1 mice. This was another flawed study, especially since its stated purpose was to replicate Sugiura's methods and to thereby test his claims.

Unlike Sugiura, who gave injections six days a week until the death of the animals, the Catholic Medical Center group gave daily injections (minus Sundays) only until the 46th day of the experiment. Mice were subsequently left untreated, and then sacrificed when their primary tumors reached a weight calculated to be four grams.

There were 25 CD8F1 mice in the treatment group and 24 in the control group. This is the point at which Martin's unique method of detecting metastases, the bioassay, enters the picture. In the laetrile-treated group, he said, just 5 animals had lung metastases upon gross examination. Five out of 25 would of course represent a lung metastasis rate of 20 percent by macrovisual observations, which was very similar to Sugiura's findings.

But Martin had a different calculation. He said that there were only 19 mice in the laetrile-treatment group. Why? Because six animals died and decomposed before they could be analyzed. Martin then said that an additional 13 animals had metastases as determined by his unique bioassay. So, according to him, this added up to a total of 18/19 animals, or 95 percent of laetrile-treated animals with lung metastases, a devastating total.

By contrast, in the control group, 4 of the 24 animals had metastases by macrovisual observation, while 11 showed metastases by bioassay. Martin thereby concluded that a total of 15/21, or 71.4 percent, in the control group had metastases. (Again, three animals mysteriously died and decomposed before they could be examined.)

Thus, by his tally, laetrile-treated animals had more metastases than controls.

Martin called this sort of assessment the "combined bioassay and macrovisual observation" method. In the SKI Paper, he spelled out what this meant in practice:

> *"The lung metastases were evaluated grossly; when*
> *apparently negative or questionable by macrovisual*
> *observation these lungs were put into bioassay for final*
> *determination of the presence of lung metastases" (p. 112).*

Please note carefully what is being said here. Any abnormality detected via macrovisual examination was accepted forthwith as positive for metastases. There was no need, Martin was saying, for microscopic confirmation that a suspicious lesion was truly cancerous. All visible abnormalities were immediately accepted as positive for cancer.

Once that was done, the lungs of all the remaining mice ("apparently negative or suspicious") were then subjected to Martin's unique bioassay.

But didn't the SKI Paper itself lecture us that macrovisual observations were "subjective determinations" that "may vary with the observer"? That they were inherently subjective and could never be accepted without further confirmation? Of course. But that was when they were making the duplicitous case that Sugiura used only such macrovisual observations to determine the presence of metastases.

Since the bioassay was itself greatly prone to false positives, Martin's "combined bioassay and macrovisual observation" method could be expected to greatly over-diagnosed the presence of lung metastases. Using such a system, one would expect both laetrile and control animals to have many perceived "metastases," so that, in the end, there would be no perceptible difference between the two groups.

And this is precisely what happened.

The percentage of mice with lung metastases was 71 percent in the control group vs. 95 percent in the laetrile group. In no case were the lungs of any of these animals subjected to microscopic examination by a professional pathologist, such as Sugiura routinely did. For all these reasons, I definitely do not think this can be accepted as a valid anti-laetrile experiment.

Second Cooperative Experiment

This experiment, like the previous one, was conducted at the Catholic Medical Center in Woodhaven (pp. 112-113). When Sugiura arrived at the Queens laboratory, he told me, Martin was nowhere to be seen. Martin, he said, left the day-to-day mouse work to technicians. Needless to say, this did not impress Sugiura, who throughout his long career was a hands-on researcher.

Although this was supposed to be a cooperative experiment, the only data given is that of Martin and his group. Macrovisually, Martin saw almost twice as many metastases in the control group as in the laetrile-treated animals. The numbers in the SKI Report are 15.4 percent in the laetrile-treated group vs. 28.6 percent in the controls. Thus, laetrile reduced the number of visible metastases in half. But Martin turned this into a negative experiment through the use of his bioassay.[284] I show elsewhere why the bioassay was an inaccurate and now thoroughly rejected method for detecting metastases. But Martin had already reached his conclusions about laetrile, and then adjusted the data to fit his preconceived prejudices.

First "Blind" Collaborative

The "First 'Blind' Collaborative Experiment is discussed on page 113 of the SKI paper. The data is given in Tables XVI and XVII on pages 114 and 115 of the paper.

Upon conclusion of the second cooperative test, a so-called "blind" collaborative experiment was begun in June 1976. In the meantime, Martin's media campaign against laetrile was in high gear. He told *Medical World News* there was not "even the remotest possibility that laetrile works."[285,286] When previously in history was any compound entrusted for testing to a scientist who knew in advance that it didn't have the "remotest possibility" of working?

When members of the New York chapter of Science for the People wrote to Dr. Good about the dangers inherent in collaborating with a man who "knew" in advance whether a putative treatment could possibly work, the SKI President replied:

> *"To my knowledge, Dr. Martin is an honest and skillful scientist.... It is natural that he should be involved in a scientific analysis concerning spontaneous tumor systems with which he has great expertise."*[287]

According to an article in the first issue of the *Second Opinion* news-letter (November 1976), the results were "quite predictable to anyone who has followed the laetrile controversy."

Sugiura was not supposed to know which mice received the laetrile and which the saline control solution. His role was simply to weigh the mice, measure their tumors and macrovisually observe their lungs, when sacrificed, for metastases.

Martin then performed his bioassay on all sacrificed mice, but neither Sugiura nor anyone else from SKI took part in this aspect of the experiment. There were certainly no microscopic examinations by independent pathologists. The whole test was therefore performed according to the idiosyncratic methods of Martin, in which the mice were sacrificed immediately after exhibiting any "growth" in the area of implantation, which would include all inflammatory and non-malignant "growths."

However, this experiment too ended in controversy, with Stock declaring that the "blindness" aspect had been lost. The SKI paper stated that this experiment

> "...*suffered a loss of assurance of blindness because of some early deaths in the [laetrile] treated group as a result of some of the injections...*" (p. 114).

Once again, Martin and his technicians had botched an experiment, accidentally killing about one-quarter of the test mice. Stock later told *Science* that the experiment "went badly because of clumsy injection procedures."[288]

But there is a huge disconnect between what the SKI paper said about this experiment and what I myself witnessed at the time it happened.

Sugiura provided me with an eight-week report on the experiment. By that point, Sugiura told me that he had guessed the "key" to the experiment. He surmised that the first set of seven cages contained the control animals and the second set of seven cages housed the laetrile-treated animals. He said that the mice in the second set of cages had a better physical appearance. Their coats were shiny, their weights were normal, they were friskier, etc. By contrast, the control animals were all moribund.

In the control cages, he said, 8 out of 35 animals, or 23 percent, experienced tumor growth stoppage as measured by his calipers. But in what he deemed to be the laetrile cages the number of tumor growth stoppages was 21 out of 34, or 62 percent (almost three times as many).

The number of new tumors in the control group was 8 out of 35, or 23 percent, while the number of new tumors in the laetrile group was just 2 out of 34, or 6 percent (almost four times fewer).

The number of lung metastases by macrovisual examination was 43 percent in the laetrile group vs. 62 percent in the controls.

It was on the basis of these parameters plus, as I said, the physical appearance of the mice, that Sugiura surmised which cohort of cages contained the treated animals and which the controls.

Elated at having figured out which mice were which, he told me that he was going to inform Stock of his deduction. In fact, he was convinced that the long struggle was over. The blind test had been completed and not only had laetrile outperformed the controls, but he had been able to correctly surmise which group was which.

From my perspective, however, I saw disaster looming. I couldn't believe how trusting Sugiura was, and I pleaded with him not to tell Stock what he surmised. Wait until the end of the experiment, I said, and then put your conclusions in a written report. But Sugiura saw no reason for trepidation, as Stock had been his trusted friend and colleague for almost 30 years.

So he told Stock his conclusions as to which animals were which, and as soon as he did, Stock abruptly called an end to the experiment! As he put it at the time, "We lost the blindness aspect."

The experiment that is published in the SKI paper bears little relationship to either Sugiura's eight-week memo or the manner in which I experienced these events unfold.

SKI later agreed that the 70 treatment and control mice were caged in a total of 14 cages and that each cage contained only laetrile-treated or saline control animals. But according to the final paper, the two types of mice were never arranged in two large discreet groups, as was stated in Sugiura's memo. Instead, the cages were supposedly arranged in a random pattern, and not possibly guessed at in the manner that Sugiura claimed.

But there is a major problem here. If this helter-skelter pattern had truly been the case, then obviously Sugiura would have been completely wrong in his eight-week assessment of which mice were which. When he reported that the mice in one discreet group of seven cages had fewer growths and metastases than in the second discreet group of cages, he would necessarily have been entirely off base. In such a case, there would have been no need to abruptly cancel the experiment.

As I wrote at the time:

> "One would think that SKI would have, at that point, announced to the world that Sugiura had 'flunked' this crucial test, and informed him of the same. Instead, Dr. Stock abruptly cancelled the experiment...and scheduled another "blind" test to take place at SKI itself. [Stock] never apparently responded to Sugiura's memos claiming 'victory.' He left Sugiura thinking he had in fact guessed correctly."[289]

I therefore conclude that the description of this experiment in the SKI report is partially fabricated, designed to cover up the fact that Sugiura had readily surmised which animals were which, based on the growth of tumors and on their physical appearance.

The Stock Challenge

The Sloan-Kettering Institute Test of Amygdalin in Spontaneous Mammary Tumors in CD8F1 Mice, is discussed on pp. 114-119 of the SKI Paper.

The final challenge to Sugiura's results came from Stock himself, in a final so-called "blind" experiment. This is the one that is most often cited by skeptics and quackbusters as "proof" that laetrile did not prevent metastases at Sloan-Kettering.

Stock's "Blind" Experiment

Despite many positive experiments at SKI, the final judgment on laetrile was relegated to another "tie-breaker" experiment. This was carried out at the Walker Laboratory. In the words of the SKI paper:

> *"It was decided to conduct a further blind test in which there would be added safeguards against a compromise of blindness in the conduct of the experiment" (p.114).*

Stock held the key to this test. The only other person who knew which mice were which was a Sloan-Kettering technician named Glenys M. Otter, who did the actual injecting.[290] Mrs. Otter (1941-2006) was a former high school teacher[291] who at that point had only appeared as a co-author on a single scientific paper.[292]

I had, and have, the greatest qualms about the integrity of this experiment. But lacking any direct evidence of fraud in this particular study, I will proceed with my analysis under the assumption that SKI's description of this study was accurate and that this was an honest attempt to replicate Sugiura's tests.

Here is how the SKI paper described this final experiment:

> *"A very carefully designed experiment with safeguards to preserve the blindness was successfully conducted. In this*

> *experiment, in which comparable readings were made of*
> *lung metastases by Sugiura and others independently*
> *without knowing the treatment the animals had received,*
> *whether AM [amygdalin, ed.] solution or saline, there were*
> *no significant differences observed between the treated and*
> *control mice."*

Stock's "greater safeguards" mainly consisted in mixing laetrile-treated and control animals in the same cages. All other researchers, including Martin, had segregated treatment and control animals in separate cages. But Stock worried that this practice had helped Sugiura to deduce which cages contained treated animals, and which contained controls. So instead, this time, treated and control animals would be mixed up in the same cages, distinguished only by earmarks, according to an international numbering code.

Stock received 84 tumor-bearing mice from Martin, which Mrs. Otter then organized into 42 matched pairs. In each pair, one mouse was to be treated with laetrile, the other injected with inert saline solution. These matched pairs were then distributed among 14 cages, with three pairs of mice per cage (three laetrile-treated and three controls per cage).

To an inexperienced outsider, this might seem like a foolproof way of conducting a totally blinded experiment. But, much to Stock's annoyance, Sugiura objected. Based on decades of practical experience, Sugiura warned Stock that there was too great a danger of the treated animals being accidentally given saline or, conversely, of the controls being given laetrile. This sort of error would compromise the final results and, under those circumstances, one would expect the final outcome in the two groups to be roughly the same.

The "earmarking" system for mice was not without pitfalls. According to the American Association for Laboratory Animal Science (AALAS):

- It is not uncommon for the holes or notches to close up over a period of time. Therefore it is important to check the markings regularly to be certain the animal can still be identified accurately.

- Errors can occur through the accidental tearing of punched earmarks or a loss of identification through biting.

- If group-housed mice fight they may rip each others' ears and cause the proper identification to be lost.[293]

Coprophagy

There is another big danger when one tries to house treated and untreated animals in the same cages. This is the problem of coprophagy. This word refers to the practice of many animals, including rodents, to eat their own feces, or the waste material of other animals. Needless to say, this is not their most attractive feature, but we must talk about it now.

"Coprophagy is an innate behavior in mice which perform it habitually,"[294] wrote one researcher. The practice actually serves a vital function by provided animals with access to vitamin B12[295] and other incompletely digested nutrients in feces. But to scientists coprophagy represents a disturbing "loss of dietary control" in their rodent experiments,[296] because it allows untreated animals to become "treated," by consuming the residue of experimental drugs in the waste of treated cagemates.

At the time of the laetrile experiments, the problem of coprophagy among caged rodents was well known to researchers. For decades, Prof. Richard H. Barnes, dean of the graduate school of nutrition at Cornell University, had warned that it could upset calculations in animal experiments.[297] There were already hundreds of articles on the topic. Since Stock was reputedly an expert on animal experimentation, he could hardly plead ignorance of the topic, nor of its wide-scale prevalence among test animals.

This problem would certainly have applied to laetrile. More recent experiments have shown that laetrile, along with half a dozen of its breakdown products (or metabolites), are excreted by animals receiving injections. This can be detected at even 1/20th the dose that Stock used in this blind experiment.[298]

Dean Barnes showed that an extraordinary 42 to 65 percent of excreted feces were later ingested by rodents, even those inhabiting cages with raised wire screen floors.[299] The implications of this for the SKI "blind" experiment is obvious: control mice were also inevitably being "treated" with laetrile and its breakdown products. As I have shown, this fact was even alluded to at the NCI Conclave in 1974, which Stock attended.

Almost as if he were referencing Stock's blind experiment, two decades earlier Dean Barnes had written:

> *"The rat can and does consume a large proportion of his fecal output even though being maintained on raised wire screens.... Many authors have commented on how this act could influence the interpretation of experimental results. In view of the assumed importance of coprophagy, it is rather surprising that so little effort has been given to its control."*[300]

Animals in Stock's laetrile experiment had ample opportunity to ingest their own, as well as their cagemates' wastes, and no effort was made to prevent this.[301]

Not surprisingly, then, the drug effects commonly seen in Sugiura's experiments with laetrile (such as temporary tumor stoppages) were seen across the entire mouse population—treated and controls—in Stock's "blind" experiment. It is safe to assume that all the animals actually received laetrile in one form of another.

Mindful of these problems, Sugiura asked Stock to house treated and control mice in separate cages, whereupon Stock could then randomize entire cages. This would have provided a sufficient degree of blindness, without the obvious difficulty of randomizing mice within cages. But Stock overruled him and the final "blind" experiment proceeded as planned.

The results, as recorded by Sugiura and other observers, showed no significant difference in metastases between laetrile-treated and control animals. Stock immediately announced this as proof that laetrile had no beneficial effect on these animals. But a more likely explanation was that they were all, to a greater or lesser degree, treated with both laetrile and saline.

In fact, Sugiura noted that there were initial tumor stoppages in 28 out of 70, or 40 percent, of the control animals vs. just 27 percent of the laetrile-treated animals. This should never have happened. As Sugiura said, with dismay, at the SKI press conference:

> *"We people in chemotherapy use saline solution because it does not stop tumor growth. Now this happens."*

Sugiura was convinced that his fears had come true and that the control animals had inadvertently received laetrile in various forms, and vice versa.

The employee group *Second Opinion* demanded an explanation of how saline-treated animals could experience more frequent growth stoppages than laetrile-treated animals. There was no answer.

It might seem at times that I was acting on my own in my investigation of Sugiura's activities. But this was not so. I was usually under the watchful eye of my immediate supervisor, Jerry Delaney. In fact, on the afternoon in July 1974 that I returned from my visit to the Walker lab, I gave Jerry a full report of my meeting with Sugiura. I told him everything that Sugiura had told me about the effects of laetrile, particularly on lung metastases in CD8F1 mice. Jerry seemed amazed, although much of what I was telling him was known from the 1973 leak. Jerry then suggested that I actively pursue my contact with Sugiura and keep him informed of whatever else I discovered.

In a broad sense, therefore, my superiors sanctioned my investigation of the laetrile experiments (although obviously I took it further than they might have wished). In addition, I was going to write an article on the life of Dr. Sugiura, so this gave me further reason to take an interest in his life, including his current activities. As it turned out, this innocent-seeming *Center News* article became a focus of concern for the administration. Either mentioning laetrile or not mentioning it was fraught with possible repercussions. After more than a year, after accumulating the comments of a dozen other administrators, the newly appointed MSKCC Executive Vice President, John D. White, scrawled on it in red ink, "Kill it!" and that was the end of the project.[302]

Keeping track of menacing controversies was of course important to the Public Affairs Department since it would have to deal with the repercussions should there be an explosion. And nothing was more volatile than laetrile. So there were good reasons that Jerry wanted to be kept informed. Of course, by doing so I also kept him informed of what I knew. He had other sources of information on Sugiura, but he had no other way of knowing about my activities in detail.

Initially, I had no thought of becoming personally involved in the controversy. I figured the issue would work itself out and, like any parent with school-age children, I already had enough on my plate. I thought I was through with any sort of political action. I was not looking for a cause and I felt alienated from the laetrile movement, which seemed dominated by the John Birch Society. The slogan "Freedom of Choice" didn't resonate with me. As I later wrote in the *Second Opinion Special Report*:

> *"Freedom of choice is not the issue. The focus of the laetrile movement should be…to demand the truth from the scientific establishment about this agent, and all issues relating to cancer."*

What drew me to the laetrile struggle were the outrageously false statements being made by the top administrators, starting with Dr. Good, and a desire to defend Dr. Sugiura, whose skill and integrity were unfairly being questioned at every turn.

My Visit to a Tijuana Clinic

Sometimes cancer patients would reach me at MSKCC, where I had become one of the *de facto* spokespersons on laetrile.[303] But what particularly impressed me was an unofficial visit to two Mexican clinics in April, 1976.

Part of my job responsibility was to accompany MSKCC scientists to meetings and help them to present their work to the media. I therefore accompanied some scientists making presentations at the 60th annual meeting of the Federation of American Societies of Experimental Biology, held that year in Anaheim, Calif.

After I had accomplished my tasks, a friend and I drove a few hours south to Tijuana, Mexico. I just showed up unannounced as an interested

American citizen. I visited the two main laetrile clinics, the Good Samaritan Hospital of Ernesto Contreras, MD and Clinica Cydel of Dr. Mario A. Soto, MD, but in neither place did I reveal my Sloan-Kettering connection.

I rambled about the premises talking to patients. I eventually got to meet Dr. Contreras. I had read a lot of negative things about him in the American media, but in person he seemed intelligent, modest in his claims, and religiously devout.

But what impressed me most were the conversations I had with American patients. Most of them had driven to Mexico under a sentence of imminent death. All the ones I met had been through grueling courses of conventional therapy or were rejecting treatments that they and their doctors agreed could not cure them. They did not want to spend their final days, as they put it, sick as a dog. I did not meet any individuals who had been duped into abandoning curative therapies back home, although of course this was just a drop-in visit, not a scientific survey.

Chemotherapy was often very harsh. It could cause distressing side effects, such as hair loss, nausea and vomiting, mouth sores, white blood cell deficiencies, and the like. Researchers had not yet come up with anti-nausea drugs that for many patients have made chemotherapy a more tolerable experience. It was bitterly ironic to many patients that laetrile was increasingly being stigmatized as 'dangerous' when back home they were being offered, in chemotherapy, some of the most toxic products ever put into the human body.

One of my interviewees, a middle-aged Midwesterner, stood out. As we sat on the edge of the fountain in the courtyard of the Cydel clinic, he said to me:

> *"When I came here I had a pain that was like"—here he gestured with the slow movement of his hand—"someone was turning a knife back and forth, back and forth in my throat. But as soon as I got here and started taking laetrile, the pain lessened. And now, a week later, it's gone."*

He looked at me with a mixture of amazement and anger, the latter directed at the federal government that had made him flee his own country in order to get this forbidden item.

Sugiura had found that, in his animal studies, even after prolonged, high-dose injectable laetrile, there was an improvement in the appearance of health and well being of the treated mice. There seemed to be a concordance between these animal studies and the anecdotal reports of palliation that I was hearing while sitting around the fountain at Clinica del Mar.

Second Opinion

ventually, in 1976, the laetrile subcommittee of Science for the People broke away and formed its own group, which we called *Second Opinion*. We intended to issue our own mimeographed newsletter. In the course of my experiences as a student activist, I had participated in creating many handmade flyers and newsletters. Even at Abraham Lincoln High School in Brooklyn, Martha and I co-edited a current events magazine called *Vanguard*, which sold not just in school but at local newsstands. At Stanford University and the University of California at Irvine, Martha and I participated in producing various underground antiwar publications. So the idea of writing, editing, laying out and distributing newsletters was neither novel nor strange to us.

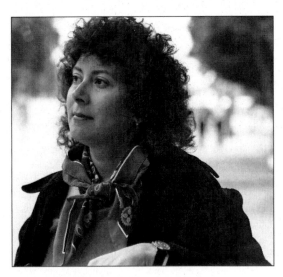

Martha Bunim Moss, circa 1977

Second Opinion functioned for the next three years and eventually published a 12-page printed newspaper, which we distributed to the 4,600 employees of MSKCC as well as to many interested outsiders.

Each quarterly edition was a big event at MSKCC. People would grab handfuls for themselves and their office mates. We were not afraid to say what was on the minds of many of the employees, who often performed difficult jobs with little recognition and insufficient pay. We found that there was more pent-up frustration at the Center than we imagined, and we became a vehicle for that discontent. Of course, we also kept the staff current on the ongoing status of laetrile testing at Sloan-Kettering.

In November 1976, *Second Opinion* made its first public appearance at MSKCC. Together with Alec Pruchnicki, Martha and I laid out the first issue of *Second Opinion* on the kitchen table of our cramped apartment in Sheepshead Bay. Later we got an office on East 3rd Street in Manhattan, between First and Second Avenues. This was an eclectic block: our near neighbors included the *Catholic Worker* magazine and the New York chapter of the Hell's Angels motorcycle club!

From the start we wanted *Second Opinion* to have mass appeal. We deliberately did not feature a story on laetrile on the first page, figuring that this might have less general interest than more locally relevant stories. Our lead articles were "SKI Student Expelled by Racist Dean," and "Cutbacks Hit MSKCC Workers." These were meant to appeal to large segments of the MSKCC community and were in fact partially written by workers and students.

Only on the inside was there a story on the laetrile controversy: "New Positive Results at SKI Squelched. Cover-Up Continues." This first laetrile article began with a concise history of the controversy:

> "Laetrile (amygdalin) is an illegal anti-cancer substance that has been in the news quite a lot lately. The people who are in favor of its use claim that it is a non-toxic vitamin, which gives pain relief in cancer, and generally stops the disease from getting worse. Those who are against it—including most of the top doctors and government health authorities— claim that is 'quackery.' A number of people who have brought laetrile into the US from Mexico, where it is made from apricot pits, have been arrested for smuggling and will soon stand trial in California."

After acknowledging Sugiura's positive results as well as the fact that others at SKI "have questioned these results," the article continued:

> *"But the SKI Administration has refused to release any of the data, favorable or unfavorable. Instead, it has conducted a four year public relations campaign, especially designed to cover-up and discredit Sugiura's results. All the real information about SKI's laetrile tests has been obtained through 'leaks' from the Institute itself."*

The article commented on the so-called "blind" test that had recently been conducted between SKI and Catholic Medical Center personnel. The article said, this test ended in a "fiasco."

This inaugural issue also contained an analysis of the power structure of MSKCC. This sort of research was something I had learned in my student-activist days at Stanford. The idea was to figure out who owned, or controlled, what. My "Bible" at the time was G. William Domhoff's classic, *Who Rules America?* Domhoff, a professor of sociology at the University of California, Santa Cruz, argued that the owners and top-level managers of large companies and foundations were the dominant figures not just in the US economy but in politics as well.

I applied that methodology to the situation at MSKCC and to the "war on cancer" in general. My rather astonishing finding was that many of the MSKCC Overseers were board members of major pharmaceutical companies, especially Bristol-Myers Squibb. This included Lewis Thomas. At the same time we tried to disavow any connection to the "narrow conspiracy theories" (as we called them) of the far right, as typified by G. Edward Griffin's 1974 book on laetrile, *World Without Cancer.*

Because of our statements about the economics of cancer, Good in 1976 accused *Second Opinion* of being "Marxists." But *Second Opinion* had no official ideology and no connections to any other political group or party. Good (unable to refute our arguments) was desperately reaching for a handy debating tool. In any case, one certainly did not have to be a Marxist to believe that giant corporations were increasingly dominating

American medicine. This proposition is far less controversial today than it was in 1976.[304]

Never ones to pull punches, *Second Opinion* baldly stated:

> *"We believe there is a cover up of laetrile at SKI and will continue to expose it, as long as valuable data remains locked in the filing cabinets of SKI, and not published openly in scientific journals."*

At the same time, I am very proud of the fact that *Second Opinion* avoided advocating or endorsing laetrile, much less getting involved in its promotion or sale:

> *"Our interest in laetrile has always been to have it be adequately tested and to have all those research results released. If it is indeed a useful agent (whether as preventive, palliative or cure) all patients should have access to it, including the poor. If it is useless, as determined by fair and extensive tests, we would oppose its use."*

Needless to say, this put us at odds with the "freedom of choice" movement, then the driving force in laetrile legalization efforts, which believed that people should be allowed to "choose their poison," regardless of scientific findings on safety and efficacy.

Here is what we wrote in our November 1976 issue:

> *"Does laetrile work? We do not know. It may turn out to be a hoax or an illusion. We are not advocating its use. But, on the other hand, we strongly urge SKI to release all of its data on laetrile, including both the positive and negative results. This will allow outside scientists to make their own judgments on this work and possibly attempt to reproduce the experiments themselves. Not to release the data, or to release it selectively, or to lump positive and negative results together, constitutes the suppression or misrepresentation of scientific work, which is intolerable."*

But the intolerable was about to happen.

The appearance of *Second Opinion* caused a sensation at MSKCC. The first issue was greeted with a sense of absolute incredulity. We had the "inside dirt" on many topics, which was no surprise since we were made up predominantly of insiders. But the fact that its authorship was anonymous, other than the mysterious front man Alec Pruchnicki of the Bronx, was maddening to Institute officials. Good commented on this at the press conference, saying rather ominously that he'd like to know who was behind it. Who were these spies, infiltrators and leakers? This was, of course, particularly troubling to me, since I knew that eventually the trail would lead to me.

We distributed the paper in the wee hours of the morning, when the night shift got off and the morning workers, including the day nurses, arrived. The distributors were all "outside agitators," colleagues from our group (some of whom, like Alec, came from Science for the People) as well as Martha and members of our family. The entire hospital seemed quiet on distribution days, as many people, including top administrators, pored over the latest issue.

But, even in those pre-Internet days, I believe that my connection to *Second Opinion* would ultimately have been traced. Sugiura had already told Stock that he had given me a copy of his lab notes. So I was definitely on thin ice. But I had made my decision and I was never going back to business-as-usual as long as the laetrile cover-up continued.

Dinner with Good

The high point in my relationship with Dr. Good came in the winter of 1976, when we dined together at New York's swanky 21 Club. The public affairs director of a large German pharmaceutical company had come to town and for reasons of his own wanted to meet the famous Robert A. Good. I had no particular interest in helping him (not least because his company was a successor to the notorious Nazi-era I.G. Farben chemical company), but I saw an opportunity to have some quality time with the Director. I wanted to find out what he really thought about a number of things, including of course laetrile.

So, with Jerry's agreement, I asked Good if he wanted to go to a dinner and a Broadway show with the visiting Germans...and me. It was a long shot and I was happily surprised when he said yes. Once we got to the restaurant we sat next to each other and then more or less ignored the Germans for a couple of hours.

As part of my personal campaign to confront the leadership over their laetrile misstatements, I used this opportunity to raise the laetrile issue with the Director. But he only spoke in platitudes on this topic and seemed disinterested.

Good was genuinely excited by other things and had an urgent desire to have those stories told. That is where I came in. He had been among the first American scientists to tour China in the post-Nixon era. We discussed co-authoring a book about his travels in China, but of course that and many other plans soon fell by the wayside.

During dinner (out of earshot of the Germans) he gently but pointedly said to me, "I am just like you, Ralph. You can be fired, and I can be fired, too." This 'prophecy' came true sooner than either of us could have realized.

Incidentally, the next day, the German official offered me $1,000 cash under the table for having so ably arranged this meeting. When I turned it down, he offered me $2,000 "but no more," he added, gruffly. I rebuffed him on this as well, but I did get an insight into the ways the pharmaceutical industry spread its influence, or at least the way it did so in 1976.

Visit from Laetrilists

In late 1976 I received an unexpected visit from three of the top officials of the Committee for Freedom of Choice in Cancer, Inc., based in Los Altos, CA. Michael Culbert, Maureen Salaman and Robert Bradford. had come to New York City on an exploratory expedition, trying to locate the source of the leaks at Sloan-Kettering. They had no appointment and no contacts but simply went to the reception desk of the hospital, asking questions about the laetrile testing. Ultimately, they were directed to my office—not because the receptionists suspected me of being the source of the leak, but because I was the Public Affairs officer whose bailiwick included non-conventional treatments. In fact, I was told that MSKCC's telephone operators had sticky notes attached to their consoles reading, "Laetrile calls go to Dr. Moss in Public Affairs."

The four of us had a strange conversation indeed. A new issue of the *Second Opinion* newsletter had been distributed that very morning and I quickly hid my copy under my IBM Selectric as they crowded into my small office. But Culbert, the brightest of the three, noticed a copy of Max Gerson's unorthodox diet-and-cancer book, *A Cancer Therapy: 50 Cases*, on my bookshelf. He shot me a quizzical look.

Bradford and Salaman looked particularly uncomfortable. They had created a bogeyman out of MSKCC and they looked as if they were ready to flee at any moment. Culbert and I later became friends and he told me that they strongly suspected that they had located the source of the leak… namely, me.

In February 1977, *Second Opinion* published another issue. We again highlighted issues of racism and class discrimination at the Center. Memorial Hospital "Admissions Biased, Racist" and "Wu's Case Stirs Action" were our front-page stories. Again, the laetrile article was relegated to page three.

At this time, Federal Judge Luther Bohanon, as part of a ruling that legalized the use of laetrile by patients for their individual use, had ordered the FDA to hold public hearings. These took place on May 2, 1977 in Kansas City. Stock appeared on behalf of SKI. His assignment was to refute the charge that Sloan-Kettering was covering up Sugiura's positive results.

It was well enough for Good, Martin and Thomas to make outrageous statements that denied the simplest facts about the testing program. But this Kansas City hearing was going to be filled with ardent and generally well-informed laetrilists. They certainly knew about the leaks from Sugiura's laboratory. Stock knew that, in that company, he could hardly deny that Sugiura had ever achieved positive results in animal systems. At the same time, with high-placed anti-laetrilists breathing down his back, he could not very well confirm these either. So this is what he said:

> *"Early observations of Sugiura featured an apparent*
> *inhibition of the appearance of metastases in the lungs of*
> *mice given daily doses of amygdalin."*

Second Opinion promptly took him to task for this:

> "*Apparent inhibition? Dr. Stock is Dr. Sugiura's immediate boss and he also heads the Walker Laboratory, where most of the laetrile experiments took place. Can't he tell us in fact whether or not the mice that received the laetrile had less [sic] secondary tumors than the controls? Didn't he look with his own eyes while the experiment was in progress? We believe he did.*"[305]

Stock had been given the delicate task of phrasing things so that they appeared credible to a scientifically sophisticated audience. He needed to create a scientific fig leaf for the cover-up. Stock continued in his FDA Affidavit:

> "*In [Sugiura's] three initial experiments the treated mice showed lung metastases in 20 percent, while 80 percent of the controls had metastases...Subsequent experiments showed that the initial results were not consistently observable.*"

This was finely worded. We'll leave aside the fact that Sugiura had performed six consecutive CD8F1 treatment experiments, not three, all of which showed marked inhibition of metastases. *Second Opinion* noted at the time:

> "*Stock constantly tries to whittle down the number of positive experiments.*"

But the essence of what he was saying was actually true. It was also true that "subsequent experiments" did not "consistently" confirm these results. For the reasons already given, Schmid, Stockert and Martin did not consistently report positive results in all their experiments. But what Stock failed to mention was that in the one experiment that really rose to the level of a genuine confirmatory study, the Schmid-Sugiura Collaborative Test, results were positive in both Schmid and Sugiura's macrovisual observations as well as, most importantly, in the independent pathologists' report.

Two months later, In April 1977 *Second Opinion* published its third issue. This time we had a front-page article on the topic that interested me most: "Laetrile: Publish or Perish."

This reported that SKI officials had completed "the latest, and probably the last, animal test with laetrile (amygdalin) at the Sloan-Kettering Institute." That was correct, since no further test has been done there, even to this day.

"According to SKI officials," *Second Opinion* wrote,

> *"This latest test does not confirm earlier findings that laetrile inhibited cancer growth, stopped the spread of cancer, and improved the health and well-being of mice. This conclusion would seem to doom the controversial anti-cancer 'vitamin,' which has been tested for over four years. But no sooner had SKI announced the alleged failure than the new study was plunged into controversy."*

As we explained in *Second Opinion*, Sugiura immediately contested the results, an unprecedented act of defiance on his part, after almost 60 years at the institution. He told reporter Mort Young of the *San Francisco Examiner* that "the tests were not done to my satisfaction." He told colleagues at the Walker Laboratory that he would stick by his earlier findings that "laetrile prevents metastases" or secondary growths in mice.

The SKI Press Conference

June 1977 was a turning point for laetrile at Sloan-Kettering. The assault on laetrile began with a blistering op-ed in the *New York Times* titled "Laetrile: A 'Fraud.'" Responding to the legalization of laetrile in two dozen states, Daniel Martin pulled out all the stops:

> *"State governments are being manipulated to legalize the quack cancer nostrum laetrile...worthless product... unproved drug...danger...deception... illusion... propaganda being propagated by laetrile's promoters...."*

Laetrile use, he continued, victimized huge swaths of the population:

> *"...the uninformed, the naïve, the innocent, the cultists, the gullibles, the fanatics, the poor, the very young, and the desperately sick...."*[306]

This diatribe set the stage for Memorial Sloan-Kettering Cancer Center's press conference. June 15, 1977 dawned as a bright, balmy day on Manhattan's Upper East Side. Within MSKCC, almost 100 reporters and observers and half a dozen film crews from the leading television stations had assembled to hear the long-awaited verdict on the unconventional treatment from doctors at the world's most prestigious cancer research center.

On the dais of the new conference room sat men and women whose credentials in the scientific world, and even among the public, were impeccable: Robert A. Good, Lewis Thomas, MD, Daniel Martin and eight other Memorial Sloan-Kettering scientists (C. Chester Stock, PhD, Kanematsu Sugiura, DSc, Isabel M. Mountain, PhD, Elizabeth Stockert, D d'Univ., Franz A. Schmid, DV., George S. Tarnowski, MD, Dorris J. Hutchison, PhD, and Morris N. Teller, PhD).

Conspicuously absent was Lloyd J. Old, who had enthusiastically launched the laetrile experiments in spontaneous tumors and had asked Sugiura to do the tests. When I first visited Sugiura in July 1974 he told me "Dr. Old believes in my results." Old convened the laetrile meetings at SKI, brought in the top practitioners and experts, and was the driving spirit behind the confidential meetings at FDA headquarters in 1974 and at NCI in 1975. But as time progressed, he disassociated himself from the controversy and made his last public comment in *Medical World News* in 1975.[307] I don't know if he was told to recuse himself or decided to do so on his own accord. The bottom line was that he did not publicly defend Sugiura.

But at least he, unlike the other top leaders, refused to make blatantly false statements about the outcome of his tests. At the time of the Press Conference, Old simply absented himself. His office let out that he was traveling in some inaccessible place—I think they actually said Tahiti!—and could not be reached for comment.

Old could have supported Sugiura in word and deed. But he knew that he would have to pay a heavy price for doing so—perhaps even losing his academic future, the way a comparable figure, Andrew Conway Ivy, MD (1893-1978), past president of the American Physiology Society and vice-chancellor of the University of Illinois, had lost his reputation over Krebiozen a decade before. So he simply made himself inaccessible on that fateful day.

Besides *Second Opinion's* attempts to support him, Sugiura had to fight on alone. All of the Sloan-Kettering leaders agreed, apparently, in the words of the official press release, that, after almost five years of testing, "laetrile was found to possess neither preventive, nor tumor-regressant, nor anti-metastatic, nor curative anticancer activity."[308]

The press conference was intended to put an end to the laetrile controversy at Sloan-Kettering and to prepare the way for Lewis Thomas' testimony before Senator Kennedy's subcommittee hearings the following month.

Officials of the center cleared their throats; reporters put down their danishes and coffee and picked up their pencils. Dr. Good began to speak. After general remarks condemning laetrile and its use, he passed the microphone to Chester Stock.

In a voice sometimes shaking with nervousness, Stock repeated Sugiura's findings, almost word for word from Sugiura's memos. This was part of the deal that had brought Sugiura himself to that very conference table.

Stock said the following (which I have transcribed from raw video footage that NBC and others took that day):

> *"Laetrile is not curative, but is a palliative agent. He [Sugiura, ed.] bases this on his own observations, reported with his experiments, which include inhibition of lung metastases, temporary initial stoppage of growth of small primaries, inhibition of the appearance of new tumors, and better health and appearance of treated mice. And this was a statement that Dr. Sugiura approved for this publication."*[309]

Sugiura, perhaps invoking some of the techniques he had learned as a martial artist, had skillfully extracted a promise from Sloan-Kettering to include all of his most pertinent findings in the final report, and of having Stock then recite these verbatim in his presentation. In the raw footage of the press conference one can see Stock leaning over the table to catch Sugiura's eye—as if to say, "Look, I did exactly as you asked."

Stock continued to explain some fine details of laetrile testing, but as his voice droned on, the eyes of many turned toward the figure on his left: a small, old Japanese scientist in a dark suit, sitting upright and impassive, blinking at the lights through thick, rimless glasses.

When the conference was thrown open for questions, someone in the audience asked the 85-year-old Member Emeritus for an explanation of his presence on the dais. This seemed, perhaps, to imply that he too now agreed with the negative verdict on laetrile.

Here is the actual dialogue with Sugiura, which was included in the CBS News feed recorded that morning:

Q. Dr. Sugiura, do you agree with the conclusions in the summary statement?

A. Which conclusions?

Q. To the effect that laetrile does not either cure or prevent cancer?

A. I agree. Of course my results don't agree (smiling nervously) but Iagree with what our Institute says.

Q. Why, if your results don't agree?

A. I don't know why but I think...

Q. (Interrupting him): Doctor, do you stick by your results?

A. Yes, I stick! I hope somebody is able to confirm my results later on.

Q. Have any other of your results ever been disputed before in the 40years that you've been here?

A. I'm here almost 60 years. Nobody disputes my work. Every paper I sent to publication has always been accepted.

Q. Why not this one then?

A. These results also were accepted for publication.... I'm hoping that somebody is able to confirm my results.

What then followed was an hour-long attempt by Stock to undermine everything that Sugiura had found in his years of meticulously documented testing. I have since attended many press conferences but cannot remember any that remotely resembled this one. I would venture to say that it was an unprecedented occurrence in the history of science: a major media event called to refute a scientist who was himself sitting on the dais, and who disagreed with the main premise of the conference itself!

One reporter then questioned Stock:

Q. Don't you think that there are further studies that are warranted.

A. We don't see any further experiments that we should conduct....All those agents that are effective in the treatment of cancer in man could be detected in the battery of tumor systems that I mentioned to you.

Stock then elaborated on a comparison that, at the time, was considered highly damaging to laetrile:

> "And I also might point out, as we do in the manuscript, that the spontaneous tumor system of Dr. Martin's, with which he's had so much experience, has been quite good at predicting, or could predict, it's actually confirmed that those materials that are active in breast cancer in man are effective in treating the spontaneous tumor system in the CD8F1 mouse."

This statement would soon come back to haunt him.

Good then chimed in:

"We have looked at all available methods for any evidence of anticancer activity and we have not found it. All other anticancer agents would be revealed positively."

This was an outrageous distortion of the truth. No other agents were curative against primary breast tumors in CD8F1 mice. Before the year was out, Stock would have to eat these words, in no less a venue than the *New York Times*.

Meanwhile, in the raw NBC footage of the event one can see Good fidgeting, touching his face, rolling his eyes, and glancing at his watch. To me, he was sending a clear message: "I'm too busy curing cancer to bother with this nonsense!"

When it came his turn to speak he said, in his foghorn voice:

"With respect to this compound and the evidence from all of these studies that we have, we would certainly not take any other compound to clinical trial. There's another issue here that is not scientific. And I think that this might justify a clinical trial. It is not possible to evaluate critically the influence on pain or well being on experimental animals. The anti-cancer influence can be evaluated."

Judging from its impact on reporters, the Public Affairs Department had accomplished its job. Only two reporters asked to see the actual paper under discussion, while the rest contented themselves with the press release. The media swallowed the idea that Sugiura's results had been successfully refuted. *Time* magazine's coverage typified the general agreement that laetrile had flunked its test at SKI:

"After five years of exhaustive studies with mice, researchers at this world-renowned institute concluded that in spite of early indications it might control the spread of tumors, the controversial drug laetrile showed no anticancer properties."[310]

Essentially, it was all over on the scientific level. The prestige of Sloan-Kettering had been thrown into the balance against laetrile, and (barring the unlikely event of a positive human trial) it was all over but the shouting. All that remained was to mop up the laetrile movement at the federal level.

The Kennedy Hearing

One might wonder why Sloan-Kettering, which did not actually publish its laetrile paper until February 1978, felt compelled to hold a press conference about it eight months earlier. The reason was that Lewis Thomas was scheduled to testify before Senator Edward Kennedy's Subcommittee on Health and Scientific Research in favor of "Banning of the Drug Laetrile from Interstate Commerce by FDA."

It would have been embarrassing in the extreme if the pro-laetrile side, whose top leaders were also invited to testify, had been able to present unpublished—and apparently suppressed—documents from Sloan-Kettering showing that laetrile was effective in stopping the spread of cancer.

When Nicholas Wade of *Science* magazine asked Daniel Martin if the laetrile tests weren't addressed to scientists, the latter blurted out:

> *"Oh, nonsense. Of course this was done to help people like [Benno] Schmidt and Congressmen answer the laetrilists."*[311]

The Kennedy hearings were an unprecedented face-to-face showdown between the pro- and anti-laetrile forces after 25 years of skirmishes. Science writer Lee Edson called it "The Great Confrontation—the Cancer Establishment vs. the Unorthodox Healers."[312] In one sense, it was a great victory for the laetrilists, who by dint of grassroots organizing had forced "the establishment" to deal with them as equals on the national stage. But by and large they were mocked and discredited once they got there.

Thomas came armed with a strongly worded and well-publicized anti-laetrile statement to answer the laetrilists. His limpid prose style was put at the service of suppressing an unwanted therapy.

Thomas told the senators:

> *"There is not a particle of scientific evidence to suggest that laetrile possesses any anticancer properties at all. I am not aware of any scientific papers, published in any of the world's accredited journals of medical science, presenting data in support of the substance, although there are several papers,*

> *one of these recently made public by Sloan-Kettering*
> *Institute, reporting the complete absence of anticancer*
> *properties in a variety of experimental animals."*[313]

Not a particle, mind you. Four years' worth of positive testing by SKI's most experienced researcher apparently did not constitute a single iota of scientific evidence in laetrile's favor. SKI's transformation from the open-minded center of fair testing to a bastion of negativity was now complete.

In his prepared statement Thomas did not even mention Sugiura's work. Only under questioning by Senator Richard Schweiker (R-PA) did Thomas concede that "it did seem in Dr. Sugiura's experiment [that laetrile] would inhibit the number of metastatic lesions in the lung." But he quickly added that the number of mice involved in these tests was "small" and that this observation was made only on "two or three occasions."

This was of course untrue. Sugiura made his observations in nine separate experiments, six CD8F1 treatment experiments, one CD8F1 prevention (prophylaxis) experiment, one AKR leukemia experiment and one Swiss Albino mouse experiment. As to the size of the experiments, we had this to say in our 1977 *Second Opinion Special Report*:

> *"The studies would have undoubtedly been strengthened had*
> *there been more mice in the experiments....But this was*
> *limited by factors beyond Sugiura's control: a lack of CD8F1*
> *mice, which are supplied by Dr. Martin under a National*
> *Cancer Institute contract."*[314]

Martin had received $1 million from the NCI to breed 3,000 CD8F1 mice. The rationale for the contract was that they were to be used in SKI's laetrile experiments. Now we learned that too few mice were available to be meaningful. One wonders where the $1 million went? If Sugiura's animal studies were insufficient to yield meaningful results, why didn't Stock ask Martin to supply the necessary quantity? In fact, Sugiura's first six CD8F1 treatment experiments involved a total of 150 mice (pp. 93-98). By contrast, some of Thomas' own experiments involved only a dozen or so rodents at a time.[315,316] Apparently, size only became an issue when laetrile was involved.

Getting Fired

I spent my spare time in the summer of 1977 at the Cornell Medical School library, across the street from Memorial Hospital, preparing the *Second Opinion Special Report* on SKI's laetrile paper. I wanted to present the public with a thoroughly accurate account of what had happened at SKI—the real story, not the ginned up version that SKI had issued.

In the fall, when a draft of the 48-page *Special Report* was completed, I met with the editors of *The Sciences,* and got a verbal agreement from them to do their own exposé of the SKI paper. After extensive peer review, *Second Opinion* printed its report and prepared to circulate it. The contact person, as always for *Second Opinion* publications, was Alec Pruchnicki. Because we feared reprisals from the institution, we chose the only member who was not affiliated with SKI.

I had a meeting at the Manhattan home of a free-lance science writer with an interest in laetrile, Robert G. Houston. Present on that occasion was one of the few East Coast doctors using laetrile, Michael B. Schachter, MD. Schachter confounded the image of the irresponsible "quack." He was a *magna cum laude* graduate of Columbia College and a 1965 graduate of Columbia's College of Physicians & Surgeons, New York. Schachter helped me with some of the scientific issues regarding laetrile's mode of action (as they were then understood). It might be of interest that for the past 35 years he has directed the Schachter Center for Complementary Medicine in Suffern, NY and is President Emeritus of the American College for Advancement in Medicine (ACAM).

We sent copies of the report to almost all of the reporters who, over the years, had expressed an interest in the laetrile situation at SKI. We also sent copies, with a personal note, to the Overseers, including the three most influential, Laurance Rockefeller, Benno Schmidt, and the chief Scientific Advisor, Sir Peter Medawar. We waited for a reaction but never heard from a single one of them.

I made a point of hanging around Jerry Delaney's office that day, as the first responses came in. A typical conversation went something like this:

Reporter: "Who's behind this *Second Opinion Special Report?*"

Jerry: "I have no idea."

Reporter: "Then, who is this Alec Pruchnicki?"

Jerry: "No idea. We've checked. He never worked at our institution."

Reporter: "Thank you for your time."

We also announced that *Second Opinion* would hold a press conference at the New York Hilton on the following day to unveil and discuss the report.

I went home that evening feeling rather sick at heart. But my son, Ben, who was just 10 years old, was literally sick that day, running a fever of 104.5° F. He saw my agitation and asked me what the problem was. I explained as best I could.

Ben said to me, "Dad, you can't go on working for them and against them for ever." He had more wisdom at 10 than I had at 34!

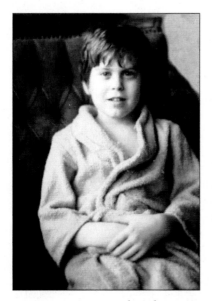 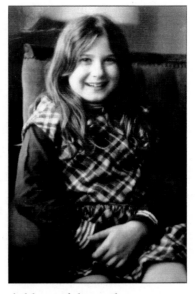

Benjamin Moss and Melissa Moss, children of the author, 1977

I discussed the situation with my family. The logic of the situation was inescapable. I had to stand up and take my share of responsibility for *Second Opinion*. But this meant almost certainly losing my job and all of the professional associations and valuable friendships that I had developed over nearly four years. And, technically speaking, I didn't have to. I could have let Alec take the brunt of this alone, something he was perfectly willing to do.

Just as I was contemplating these momentous questions that Thursday evening the telephone rang. It was Jerry!

"I was thinking," he said. "I'd like you to go to that *Second Opinion* meeting with a tape recorder tomorrow. Only don't announce yourself as belonging to Sloan-Kettering." In other words, I was to go as a spy to my own meeting.

"I can't do that," I said slowly, trying to think my way out of this dilemma.

"How come?"

"Because…ehr…I'm taking the day off tomorrow."

"You are? How come?"

"Because I'm…going to the press conference as an observer." Pause.

"Why?"

So the moment of truth had finally come.

"Because I'm going to speak at the conference on behalf of *Second Opinion*," I said. Long pause.

"I'll get back to you." He never did.[317]

That night Martha and I loaded our Chevy Impala with boxes of the *Special Report*. We parked the car in front of our apartment house to be extra safe and then spent a restless night because we knew we had to be at the press conference by 10 am. But when we went downstairs to drive into Manhattan, the Impala was gone and with it went almost our entire supply of *Special Reports*. We wound up taking a car service into the city, with a handful of the *Reports* that we had in our possession.

When we showed up at the Hilton Hotel on Sixth Avenue there were about a dozen reporters present. Mike Culbert and others from the Committee of Freedom of Choice, Inc. had latched onto our conference for their own purposes. In a moment of political naivety, we let them "co-sponsor" the event. David Leff, who attended as a reporter for *Medical World News*, explained to me how this could be used to isolate us from the mainstream media. And that is exactly what happened. In fact, sad to say, David was in the lead in doing so in his own journal! Luckily, not every reporter saw things this way, and in time the story made headlines.

I spoke first, explained who I was, outlining our position and what was written in our *Special Report.* But of course most of the interest was in the fact that I was an employee of Sloan-Kettering. This finally explained how *Second Opinion* came about, and how we knew so much about the inner workings of the Institute.

I explained the fallacies in the SKI study, as I have done in this book. The reporters seemed generally neutral. I could understand their ambivalence. It was one thing to claim positive results, but quite another to butt heads with the most powerful cancer hospital in the United States. Yet here I was unambiguously calling top Sloan-Kettering executives liars. News of my disclosure was carried on the front page of the *New York Post,* but there was no mention in the *New York Times* until one week later, on November 24, 1977, which happened to be Thanksgiving, one of the slowest news days of the year.[318]

On the Sunday after the *Second Opinion* news conference I spoke at a meeting of the National Health Federation (NHF) at the Roosevelt Hotel in Manhattan. There were over 1,000 people in attendance and I got a rousing reception from this pro-laetrile crowd.

I don't know what I expected, but when I showed up for work on Monday morning I did not receive such a tumultuous reception. I was called into Jerry's office and summarily fired. Jerry did not argue; he just gave me my walking papers.

Some of the language of what he said was preserved in his response to the *New York Times* on my firing:

> "Mr. Moss was discharged 'because he betrayed the trust
> placed in him as a member of the public affairs department
> of this cancer center. By declaring himself an author and
> spokesman for the group [Second Opinion, ed.], which
> stands in outspoken opposition to the most fundamental
> principles and policies of this cancer center, he has acted in a

*manner that conflicts with his most fundamental job
responsibilities.*"[319]

Of course I shouldn't have expected anything else but, inexplicably, I started crying. Not bawling, but definitely tears! I can't explain this except to say that at some level I must have clung to some faith in the institution. Subconsciously, I expected someone (Benno Schmidt? Laurance Rockefeller?) to order an investigation, in which the truth would finally come out. That is the way things happened in a Frank Capra movie, but in real life they tell you to find a cardboard box and clear out your office within the hour.

My fellow employees, who had supported me in my showdown with Stock in the previous year, now avoided my glance. I experienced the ostracism that often follows a firing. Of course, open mutiny and insubordination against the "company" were dangerous. Only one person offered to help me assemble my stuff: Jerry Delaney's secretary, Stanley Smith.

Soon after I was fired, I ran into Chester Stock as we hurried in opposite directions in the corridor between the old and new hospitals.

"I've been fired," I said, still in a state of shock.

"Good riddance!" he shot back. He seemed to take a bitter enjoyment from my misfortune.

Not knowing what to say I mumbled something about writing a book about my experiences. I had been working in a desultory way on a history of cancer research, but, oddly, the idea of writing a book on the "cancer industry" (as I later called it) only came to me as a feeble comeback line at the moment of my firing.

In my office, my filing cabinet had been chained and padlocked. I was told to come back in a few days later to dispose of its contents. This led to an almost surrealistic scene as I was summoned to the office of Charlie Forbes, the MSKCC vice president (and Jerry's boss), who had formally been responsible for hiring me. We always got along well. He and I opened the chained filing cabinet together and then one by one he held up a file and we discussed its disposition. Some of these files he let me keep; others, for no apparent reason, he decided to retain. Since my decision to step forward at the *Second Opinion* press conference had been last minute, I foolishly had failed to make photocopies of many relevant documents. This omission was to come back to haunt me.

After I said goodbye to Charlie Forbes (who seemed inexplicably friendly), two guards escorted me to the 68th St. exit of the building. One of them, his hand resting on his sidearm, told me never to enter the building again. It was chilling.

The radio show host Gary Null, who had an alternative medicine-oriented show on WABC, somehow learned about my firing before I had even finished packing up my office. My firing then became a *cause célèbre* for him and I appeared several times on his show. Null began an energetic on-air campaign to get Sloan-Kettering officials to formally respond to my charges. At first, Stock derisively said he would not enter into a "pissing contest with a skunk." A few weeks later, however, the story of my firing continued to generate bad publicity for SKI and didn't show any signs of going away. So SKI finally agreed to have Stock appear opposite me on Gary Null's show.

Stock and his entourage swept into the cramped studio. I was seated in another, with a thick glass wall between us. We glowered at each other. I started by explaining to the audience that Sloan-Kettering was refusing to appear in the same room with me, and that although I could see them I could not actually talk to them. On air, I compared this to something that many New Yorkers remembered: the time that a Palestinian delegation had refused to appear in the same TV studio as Israeli representatives.

Debating Stock was both enjoyable and easy. The whole thing turned out to be a public relations disaster for MSKCC.

The day after I was fired Alec checked our post office box in the Bronx and found the following letter waiting for us:

> "I wish to thank you very much for the copy of your paper entitled, Second Opinion Special Report: Laetrile at Sloan-Kettering, November 16, 1977, which you so kindly sent to me last week. I read your paper in the monograph with great interest. Your critical review of my positive results and negative results of 3 investigators at Sloan-Kettering Institute is very well done and accurate. Please accept my sincere congratulations."

It was signed "Kanematsu Sugiura."

In a sense, that made the whole ordeal worthwhile.

In April 1978, Stock, emboldened by the "successful" publication of the SKI paper, decided to take a hard line towards all further inquiries. For instance, he refused to cooperate with Rep. John T. Kelsey, Democrat of Michigan, who inquired about inconsistencies in SKI's laetrile studies. He wrote in an irascible tone:

> *"We have devoted more time to amygdalin than has been justified. I am no longer willing to request my associates to take time from current studies to answer your endless questions nor do I intend to do so myself."[320]*

The last reporter to speak to Sugiura was Gabe Pressman, then working for WNEW-TV in New York City. On May 16, 1979, Sugiura ruefully told Pressman:

> *"I am not allowed to talk about laetrile."[321]*

Sugiura continued to work up until several weeks before his death from a stroke on October 21, 1979. He was 87 years of age. That was the effective end of the laetrile saga at Sloan-Kettering.

Bob Good's dismissal from Sloan-Kettering was almost as sudden as my own. In the late 1970s, Lewis Thomas came down with a cancer-like blood syndrome, and in 1980 was replaced as MSKCC President by Paul Marks, MD. Author Philip Boffey recalled in a *New York Times Magazine* article:

> *"Key board members held Good responsible for the painted-mouse scandal and for creating the atmosphere in which a scientist would resort to cheating. Marks at first told Good that he could stay on as a tenured senior scientist, and Good accepted. But as months went by, Good found his scientific accomplishments denigrated or ignored. Good lost his spacious office. His laboratory was moved into smaller quarters. Budgets for his favored research projects in immunology were cut. Although Marks denies it, others say he asked Good to leave."*

It was a time of great bitterness, although Good never went public with his disappointment and was able to negotiate a settlement for himself.[322] He eventually landed a congenial job as Physician-in-Chief of All Children's Hospital in St. Petersburg, Florida, and Distinguished Research Professor at the University of South Florida. But of course his glory days as leader of the War on Cancer were behind him.[323]

In 1970, Good had won the Lasker Clinical Research Award "for his uniquely important contributions to our understanding of the mechanism of immunity," which put him on track for the Nobel Prize. But the Summerlin Affair had killed his chances of winning a Nobel. In 1980 Baruj Benacerraf and two others won the Nobel Prize that many people felt should have also recognized Good's epochal achievements. He had to content himself with a brief mention in Benacerraf's acceptance speech.

Good died on June 13, 2003 at the age of 81. When I learned that he had esophageal cancer, I wrote him a sympathetic note, offering to help in whatever way I could. But he never replied.

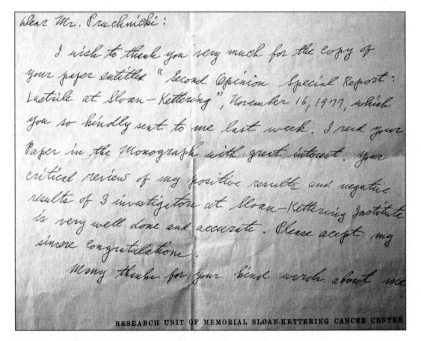

Excerpt of Sugiura's letter of November 22, 1977

Is Cancer Curable in CD8F1 Mice?

We now must return to an issue that was raised by the original SKI laetrile report. Although far from the biggest lie in the report, this was the only one that grabbed the attention of the mainstream media. It embarrassed MSKCC leaders for a short time, but was soon forgotten. In fact, instead of punishing Martin, they rewarded him with a research position at Sloan-Kettering!

In the version of the paper released at the SKI Press Conference, they claimed that primary tumors in CD8F1 mice could be cured through the use of drugs that were normally employed in the treatment of human cancer.

Assuming that laetrile had been proven through their experiments to be totally inert, it was then compared unfavorably to standard "curative" drugs. Much was made of this comparison. The original paper stated unequivocally:

> "Of those 8 agents declared clinically active against human
> breast cancer by the National Cancer Institute, all 8 agents
> also are active against this murine [mouse, ed.] breast
> cancer...Thus, the negative laetrile findings in this animal
> tumor model appear particularly significant."

This seemed damning. Even if one believed, as I did, that Sugiura's work was valid regarding the prevention of metastases, still laetrile had been conspicuously unable to cure established tumors. But in the summer of 1977, I undertook a closer examination of the SKI paper in preparation for writing the *Second Opinion Special Report*. This led me to examine Martin's earlier papers on the topic and I was very surprised to discover that the truth was exactly the opposite of what the paper stated. When used against primary tumors in CD8F1 mice, in the way that laetrile had been tested, no drug was curative. A few could possibly shrink about 20 percent of tumors, but none came close to curing the disease. None! Everything hinged on the words "clinically active." This meant only minor and temporary shrinkages of some tumors for a few weeks' duration.

No one knew this better than Daniel Martin. As early as 1957, Martin (writing under his birth name, Daniel M. Shapiro) had noted that agents that worked in the laboratory against transplanted tumors did not typically work against human tumors.

"A number of chemotherapeutic agents which have effected 'cures' of solid experimental [transplanted, ed.] tumors in the laboratory have had essentially no effect on a variety of solid tumors in the clinic [among humans, ed.].... This divergence in response has not yet been explicable and has led to grave concern over the possibility of fundamental differences between spontaneous and transplanted tumors."[324]

That was the reason that he had turned to the study of spontaneous tumors, and had developed the CD8F1 mouse in the first place, in the hope of finding a more predictive tumor model. But as it turned out chemotherapy did not work much better in these, either.[325]

So, in 1964, Martin proposed an ingenious solution to the difficulty of curing spontaneous tumors in mice. He wrote:

> *"We have found that maximal effects of chemotherapy are*
> *obtained when the bulk of tumor tissue is removed*
> *surgically, prior to the administration of chemotherapy."*[326]

To be clear, Martin first physically excised the animal's primary tumor, and then used chemotherapy, but only as an adjuvant (or additive) treatment. Alternately, he would remove a tumor from a female mouse and transplant it into a corresponding male mouse. In either case, it was only under these artificial circumstances that chemotherapy could be made to have any appreciable effect against a spontaneous tumor in CD8F1 mice.

Martin summarized the situation with CD8F1 in 1970:

> *"Nineteen chemotherapeutic compounds and two*
> *non-specific immunity-stimulating agents have been studied*
> *at length as to their effectiveness in the treatment of this*
> *tumor. Spontaneous mammary cancers in mice have proved*
> *to be quite resistant to influence by chemotherapy alone.*

> *Such anti-cancer agents as uracil mustard, Endoxan,*
> *5-mercaptopurine and thioguanine, as well as many others*
> *which have been shown to influence the growth of*
> *transplanted tumors, have been ineffective in this*
> *spontaneous tumor system.*"[327]

Only one drug, cyclophosphamide (Cytoxan), yielded temporary and/ or partial remissions in this system. In 1975, after more than a decade of disappointments, Martin concluded:

> *"Evaluation against spontaneous mammary tumors in their*
> *autochthonous hosts is the most rigorous test system...."*

"Autochthonous" in this context means that the tumor is still growing in the animal in which it first arose, and not excised or transplanted into a different animal. Martin continued:

> *"Cure has thus far been impossible to achieve by*
> *chemotherapy alone on large primary tumors. Hence, this*
> *most difficult methodology has been largely shelved in favor*
> *of evaluation by combined modality therapy, i.e., in*
> *conjunction with the surgical reduction of primary*
> *tumors."*[328]

This was the statement that caught my attention in the summer of 1977 and eventually led to a huge embarrassment for SKI. Any well-informed scientist in the field, including Stock, should have been aware of this key characteristic of spontaneous breast tumors in mice. In fact, Sloan-Kettering had done some of the original studies on this topic.

But when the *Second Opinion Special Report*, in November 1977, exposed the incurability of primary tumors in CD8F1 mice, Stock expressed astonishment. He knew nothing about it, he said. Martin had deceived him.

It then became clear that SKI had tested laetrile using a methodology that had been "largely shelved" for all other potential agents. Then they took it down from the shelf, as it were, to test laetrile. As I wrote, tongue in cheek, in the *Second Opinion Special Report*, "it is almost as if they wanted it to fail."

Criticism in the Scientific Media

After completing my work on the *Second Opinion Special Report* I naturally wanted to disseminate these findings to influential scientists and journalists. At the suggestion of my friend, Pat McGrady, Sr., the former science editor of the American Cancer Society, I approached editors of a magazine called *The Sciences* with a draft of the *Special Report*.

The Sciences was the award-winning publication of the New York Academy of Sciences (NYAS). Pat had worked productively in various NYAS committees. He felt that the NYAS was fair in its approach to non-conventional treatments and reasonably independent of MSKCC influence. I therefore approached the editor, Robert N. Ubell, and associate editor, Richard D. Smith. They were quite excited by the story I had to tell and prepared an article that, when published, confirmed many of *Second Opinion*'s charges.

Another scientific publication that confirmed some of our critique was *Science*. The author of that article was Nicholas Wade. Alec and I met him in November at a hotel on 42nd Street. A fellow Classicist, Wade later became a celebrated science writer and editorialist for the *New York Times*.

What most grabbed these seasoned reporters' attention was the following statement in the paper that SKI had released at the June 1977 press conference:

> "...the negative laetrile findings in this animal tumor model [CD8F1, ed.] appear particularly significant."

As Wade later wrote in *Science*:

> "Second Opinion *states, apparently with justice, that neither leg of this important argument stands up. The eight agents effective against human breast cancer are only active against the CD8F1 tumor when it is transplanted into another host, not when it is in its original host. Laetrile was tested only*

*against original host tumors, giving no basis for comparison
with the eight effective agents."*[329]

After *Second Opinion's* critique appeared, SKI dove for cover. Wade wrote:

*"Stock agrees that the statement is incorrect; in fact the drafts
of the report he now hands out have the paragraph in
question excised" (ibid.)*

This was a "key point," Wade said.

Stock attributed the error to Daniel Martin's "enthusiasm." This was one of the strangest explanations of scientific malfeasance I have ever heard. Martin's "enthusiasm," after all, was to destroy laetrile by any means necessary. One might as well say that Captain Ahab was enthusiastic about whales! Since Martin himself had exposed the incurability of primary tumors in CD8F1 mice, one can only conclude that his "enthusiasm" had led him down the path of outright deception.

We released the *Second Opinion Special Report* on November 17, 1977. On December 12, *The Sciences* issued its own news release, reiterating and amplifying our charges against Martin and SKI.

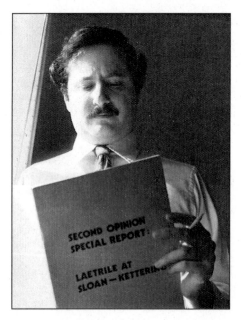

Author reviewing newly released Second Opinion Special Report, *1977*

Sloan-Kettering's laetrile paper, *The Sciences* added:

> "...*made the claim that the spontaneous tumors were susceptible to every drug known to work against human breast cancer. The claim was in error.*"[330]

Like *Science*, they revealed that SKI was hastily retracting these erroneous claims in its laetrile paper:

> "*Memorial Sloan-Kettering has backed off from a claim made in June that a particular set of laetrile experiments performed at the center over the past five years had shown the controversial apricot-derived drug to fail where conventional cancer chemotherapy had succeeded.*"

The Sciences article, which appeared in print in January 1978, disclosed:

> "*In fact the animal tumors on which the experiments in question were done are among the most drug-resistant of experimental cancers, and...many drugs that are effective against cancer in human patients have never even been tested on them.*"[331]

If one accepted the validity of Sugiura's results, then laetrile had succeeded (at least in preventing metastases) where all other drugs had failed.

The *New York Times* also publicized *Second Opinion*'s revelations, but only after attributing them to the New York Academy of Sciences. On December 13, 1977, the *Times'* medical reporter Lawrence K. Altman, MD, stated as follows:

> "*Some of the evidence from the animal testing used in a Memorial-Sloan Kettering Cancer Center report on laetrile last June has been found to be 'erroneous,' according to* The Sciences, *a magazine published by the New York Academy of Sciences...The dispute calls into question the process by which the scientific work was reported.*"[332]

As Altman wrote in the *New York Times*:

> *"The description of the tumor test system was attributed*
> *to Dr. Daniel S. Martin of the Catholic Medical Center*
> *of Brooklyn and Queens, a co-author of the Memorial*
> *Sloan-Kettering report. He said that the description was*
> *not erroneous but 'misleading' and 'not as complete as it*
> *should be.'"[333]*

Martin's hairsplitting—"erroneous," "misleading" and "incomplete"—would have been comical, had the consequences not been tragic. In an attempted exoneration of his own "misleading" statements, Stock tried to cast the blame on Martin:

> *"We accepted the statement from Dr. Martin as submitted. I*
> *did not check the original publications to be certain of the*
> *appropriateness of the statement. It should not have been*
> *used in the context of this report, and therefore it has been*
> *deleted."[334]*

This was as close as Stock ever came to a *mea culpa*. Needless to say, it is the responsibility of an author, especially a first author, to be intimately familiar with the material in his paper. But Stock could not help adding:

> *"There are no changes in the data, nor are there any*
> *retractions in the data."[335]*

This was another misdirection, since the question at hand was not about the tabulated data. In this instance, the significance of the data (not the actual results achieved) was at issue. The meaning of the paper changed, once one realized that laetrile had been tested in a system in which every other form of treatment had failed.

The New York Academy of Sciences played a mixed role in the controversy. Both Bob Ubell and Richard Smith did their own independent investigation and deserved great credit for revealing major errors in the SKI report. But Herbert J. Kayden, MD, president of the NYAS, attempted to deflect criticism from Sloan-Kettering by making Martin the "fall guy" for their combined flaws. In a rebuke to the surgeon from Queens, Kayden said:

> *"Misrepresentation by Dr. Martin was not excusable, and Dr. Stock deserves credit for correcting the error in the scientific report."*

It was satisfying to see Martin called out in public for his outrageous behavior. But, amazingly, Stock was simultaneously praised for what he also should have been reprimanded.[336] According to Kayden, Stock had saved the world from Dr. Martin's misrepresentations! In effect, Stock copped a plea of carelessness in order to fend off the much more serious charge of scientific fraud. This was very similar to what happened in the Summerlin scandal of a few years before. But this time, the main culprit was not sent to the "minor leagues" (in Summerlin's case a dermatology practice in Arkansas) but was actually promoted to a research position in the Department of Medicine of MSKCC, as soon happened to Daniel Martin.[337]

Publication of SKI Paper

When "Antitumor Tests of Amygdalin in Spontaneous Animal Tumor Systems," was finally published in the *Journal of Surgical Oncology* in February 1978 the offending statement on the curability of tumors in CD8F1 mice was indeed revised. [338] The paper conceded that drugs that worked against human breast cancer only worked when tried against tumors that had been artificially transplanted into CD8F1 mice, not against autochthonous tumors. The paper now stated:

> "In the original pre-publication version of this paper the
> paragraph making the above point did not state that the test
> system, which established the unique therapeutic
> correlations between this animal tumor and human cancer
> findings, employs first generation tumor transplants."

However laetrile was tested against "autochthonous tumors" in mice unmodified by surgery, and not against tumors that had first been transplanted.

But, in the Addendum to the final paper, the authors outrageously threw fuel on the fire. They actually reasserted what had been first been exposed by *Second Opinion* and then independently by *The Sciences*, *Science* and the *New York Times*. The irrepressible Dr. Martin once again claimed that his CD8F1 system was particular "relevant" to human cancer. At this point, Martin was not just attacking laetrile but defending the rationale for his proprietary mouse colony.

> "The CD8F1 murine [mouse, ed.] spontaneous mammary
> cancer is an animal tumor model with clinical therapeutic
> predictive ability because the anticancer agents considered
> clinically active against human breast cancer also are
> effective against this murine breast cancer."

This was false. Chemotherapy had only minor effects against auto-chthonous breast tumors in CD8F1 mice. That is why Martin had earlier written that it had been "shelved" for such evaluations. Common anti-cancer agents were only "active" in this system if their spontaneous tumors were first removed from the afflicted animal and then trans-planted into another mouse. But truly spontaneous and autochthonous tumors in CD8F1 mice could not be cured by any known means.

But the SKI paper's Addendum, whose first author was Martin, "doubled down" on its misleading claims:

> "*Therefore, in this therapeutically relevant animal tumor*
> *model, the finding that laetrile is devoid of anticancer*
> *activity is particularly pertinent*" (p. 122).

Martin was manipulating words here, in fact twisting the facts into an unrecognizable shape. CD8F1 was *not* a good model in which to test drugs against "autochthonous" tumors. Nonetheless, this is how laetrile was tested—against autochthonous tumors, not against mice that had first been surgically altered through either excision of a tumor or transplanta-tion into a different animal.

Stock, with his back to the wall, had repeatedly acknowledged the falsity of the original statement in *The Sciences, Science* and the *New York Times.* He even changed the wording of the main body of the paper to reflect this fact. But in "his" section, Martin resorted to a crude rewriting of history. It was as if the revelations of November and December 1977 had never occurred! This "particularly pertinent" comment was a complete reversal of the truth. What Martin should have said was this: "In this therapeuti-cally irrelevant animal tumor model, the supposed finding that laetrile is devoid of anticancer activity is *not* pertinent."

Thus, if laetrile did not fail in CD8F1 mice, it was much better than other agents. But even if it failed to shrink or cure tumors, this finding was irrelevant, because other chemotherapeutic agents had also inevitably failed.

Stock's public show of dismay in November at Martin's deception, and the tongue lashing the latter received from the President of the New York

Academy of Science, did not have much impact on the final paper, especially the Addendum, which turned into Martin's self-justification. In fact, Sloan-Kettering seemed impotent in the face of what Stock euphemistically called Martin's "enthusiasm."

The Addendum ascribed any confusion to *Second Opinion* and others who maliciously misrepresented the authors' crystal clear statements. About the discredited section on the relevance of CD8F1 mice, the SKI authors wrote:

> *"That paragraph placed within the context of a report on spontaneous animal tumors was interpreted by some to indicate that the therapeutic correlations were determined on the murine [mouse, ed.] spontaneous tumor system per se; therefore, that paragraph has been deleted from the paper so as not to be misleading in this regard" (p. 122).*

This was after-the-fact rationalization, because the omitted paragraph had clearly stated that laetrile had failed where other agents that were effective against human breast cancer had succeeded. In fact, autochthonous breast tumors in CD8F1 mice could never normally be cured, and the system had consequently been "shelved" (Martin's word) for further evaluations of action against spontaneous tumors. This meant that, even in the case of failure, there would be no particular relevance to laetrile's inability to cure or not cure cancers in these mice.

Therefore, at the SKI press conference, laetrile was condemned based on an out-and-out lie. We were told that laetrile had failed where other effective drugs had succeeded. But this was untrue. All other agents were, at best, only minimally effective. On the basis of this lie, however, any hopes of a scientific future for laetrile were destroyed; it was relegated to the dustbin of history.

The Aftermath

For several years after I was fired my colleagues and I kept up our campaign to disseminate the truth about SKI's laetrile testing. Alec, Martha and I, along with a changing cast of MSKCC employees, continued to publish *Second Opinion* from our Third Street office. In fact, now that I was unemployed I had more time to devote to the cause. For a while, *Second Opinion* grew in size and circulation.

I recently came across the record of a television broadcast by the TV reporter Gabe Pressman. Here is Pressman's description of our activities in May 1979:

> *"Once every couple of months, the young man and his wife appear outside the Sloan-Kettering Institute for Cancer Research on Manhattan's East Side. Ralph Moss is on a crusade denouncing what he calls a cover-up by this institution on the issue of laetrile. For three and a half years Moss worked in its Public Affairs Department of Sloan-Kettering, but he was fired in 1977, he says, because he decided to tell the truth about experiments conducted at the institution."*

After I was fired, Sloan-Kettering did all it could to undermine my ability to deliver my message. They knew that my weakest point was financial. Martha and I had very little in the bank and, additionally, Martha was unemployed at the moment. Although they had clearly fired me, they contested my right to receive unemployment insurance, claiming that I had "fired myself."

Facing an expensive and drawn-out legal process, I found an ally in Henry Rothblatt, Esq. He was a colorful Bronx-born attorney who specialized in defending "the little guy" from the "establishment Goliath."[339] This modern-day Clarence Darrow offered to take my case *pro bono;* seeing that I had obtained an aggressive and media-savvy attorney, MSKCC dropped their case.

It was significant, I felt, that although I was publicly calling them liars in every public venue to which I had access, they never threatened to sue me. Probably they were advised not to do so because they would gain little monetarily and would certainly garner a great deal of bad publicity. Henry Rothblatt would have loved a juicy public lawsuit. Or perhaps, I thought, they knew that what I was saying was true and did not want this exposed in a court of law.

I drew up a proposal for a book about cancer and Bob Ubell, editor-in-chief of *The Sciences,* volunteered to show it to several publishers, but we found no takers. I then retained a well-connected literary agent, Ruth Hagy Brod, but even she found it next to impossible to find a home for my book. One after another New York publishers turned it down, although some acknowledged that my sample chapters were well written. Larry Ashmead (1932-2010), editor-in-chief of J.B. Lippincott, asked me to co-author a less controversial popular medical book. The only one who offered to publish my cancer book was a quirky, right-wing publisher in Connecticut, whom I turned down.

In despair, I instructed Ruth to take the book off the market. "Plan B" was to do the book that Larry Ashmead had offered me. (This became *An Alternative Approach to Allergies,* which I wrote with Theron G. Randolph, MD). But, as fate would have it, that weekend Ruth attended a dinner party, where she told the other guests about the difficulties she was having getting my story in print.

One of the attendees was the CEO of a Fortune 500 company, who knew a New York publisher. Within a week I had signed a contract with Barney Rossett, founding publisher of Grove Press, and I couldn't have been happier. I had the same publisher as the Nobel laureates Samuel Beckett and Albert Camus! My editor at Grove Press was Kent Carroll, who did a superb job, helping to channel some of my raw emotions in more productive directions.

The Cancer Syndrome was published in 1980. The title was Barney Rossett's idea, influenced by the then popular movie, *The China Syndrome.* The book got many excellent reviews and I got a big boost when I received the following jacket quotation from the two-time Nobel laureate, Linus Pauling, PhD:

> *"The revelations in this book about the ways in which the American people have been betrayed by the cancer establishment, the medical profession, and the government are shocking. Everyone should know that the 'war on cancer' is largely a fraud, and that the National Cancer Institute and the American Cancer Society are derelict in their duties to the people who support them."*

I also was on *60 Minutes* in 1980, but that experience turned out to be more of a testimony to the long reach of MSKCC than of any skill on my part. A producer from *60 Minutes* had approached my agent wanting to do a segment based on *The Cancer Syndrome*. We were thrilled, as this would have put sales, already brisk, over the top. I met the producers for lunch in midtown Manhattan and we started working together on a segment, to be narrated by Harry Reasoner. However, since they had recently done a follow-up piece on laetrile, they wanted a fresh focus. Eventually they settled on the story of Lawrence Burton, PhD, a New York cancer researcher who had opened an unconventional clinic in Freeport, The Bahamas.

I was of course disappointed that the full story of laetrile at Sloan-Kettering would not be the focus of the segment. But I thought I could still provide a framework within which controversial treatments struggled for survival. I went to CBS headquarters on 57th St. at the appointed time and taped an hour-long interview. As the date approached, however, a strange thing happened. We learned that my comments, which had provided a kind of running commentary to the episode, were getting whittled down. Eventually, a three-way battle developed between my agent, the staff of *60 Minutes*, and various representatives of the "establishment." A tag team of "establishment" types kept demanding that the show be killed entirely. When *60 Minutes* producers refused to do that, these mysterious personages demanded that, at a minimum, I be removed from the segment.

Exactly who was making these demands I never found out, but it did not escape my notice that Benno Schmidt (vice-chairman of the MSKCC board) was also a director of CBS. But Ruth's husband, an aggressive stockbroker named Al Brod, had a business relationship with CBS Chairman William Paley and he assured me of my continued presence on the show. In the end, he did manage to negotiate my inclusion in the segment. When "The Establisment vs. Lawrence Burton" aired on May 18, 1980 they allotted me exactly one minute of air time.[340]

Someone quipped that they should have called that show *60 Seconds,* instead of *60 Minutes.*

My appearance did nothing for book sales, but it was not entirely a waste. The day after the segment aired I was crossing Sixth Avenue in Greenwich Village when a homeless man approached me for spare change. As I fished in my pocket, his face suddenly lit up.

"You," he said, in amazement, "You were on TV!"

Well, at least someone was paying attention.

One document that was missing at the end of my session with Charlie Forbes was official acknowledgement that my job title was Assistant Director of Public Affairs. I had been promoted to that position on my third anniversary, which was June 3, 1977, and I never imagined that documentation of this fact might ever become an issue. For the next dozen years, MSKCC readily affirmed to anyone who asked that in addition to being the science writer I had also been Assistant Director of Public Affairs at the time of my firing. Then, suddenly in 1993, after I had been appointed an advisor to the National Institutes of Health's Office of Alternative Medicine (OAM), I received a call from a reporter for the *Journal of the American Medical Association (JAMA).*

Taking a very accusatory tone, he told me that he had seen my employ-ment records and, as proof, quoted back to me my salary history. He claimed that there was no reference in my file to my being an Assistant Director of the department. According to him, I had been hired as a science writer, had been fired as a science writer, and had therefore been lying about my position all those years.

To make matters worse, he said that Jerry Delaney had told him that he had no recollection of there even being such a position as an Assistant Director.

Some time later, I ran into Jerry in Lincoln Center plaza, near where I then lived. We chatted for a while and I invited him to my apartment for coffee later that week. We spent a couple of hours "catching up" and I naturally brought up the matter of the assistant directorship. He said that he had told the *JAMA* reporter that he couldn't recall there being such a position, but that his memory in general was very poor. I remembered this to be true from my years working for him. At the time it was an amusing eccentricity, but his lack of memory had become harmful.

The more serious issue was that somebody at MSKCC had purloined my employment file and was showing it to hostile reporters. I therefore had my lawyer contact the MSKCC Administration and, as a first step, demand my right to review these same records. But access was denied, on the grounds that employee records are confidential, even from the employee himself! My lawyer reminded MSKCC that someone was already showing these records to a reporter, but they denied any knowledge of this leak.

When the *JAMA* reporter next contacted me, I demanded that he show me the documents that he had illicitly received. I informed him that he might have violated federal statutes by having possession of my personnel records. He nervously stated that he had only been shown the records, and copied the information by hand, but had never been given a physical copy. So I was being called a liar without having any way to definitively clear my name.

It took the MSKCC Administration more than 15 years, from 1977 to 1993, to decide that I was not the former Assistant Director of Public Affairs, but "merely" a science writer. Luckily, there is a good deal of evidence that I was indeed who I claimed to be.[341]

In the ensuing years, numerous reporters wrote about my case. Each contacted MSKCC to confirm my claims, starting with my job title. The list includes writers for the *New York Times*, *Science*, Associated Press, United Press International, *New York Post*, *New Scientist*, *Palm Beach Post*, *Arizona Republic*, *Denver Post*, etc. Certainly I did not simultaneously hypnotize all of these seasoned journalists into publishing a "lie" that I was Assistant Director of Public Affairs at MSKCC when I was fired.

Return to MSKCC

L loyd Old referred many cancer patients to the telephone consultation service that I began after leaving MSKCC. In 2010 he and I had a very pleasant phone conversation, during which he told me that he admired and approved of the help I gave patients struggling with wrenching decisions. Patients would tell me, in turn, of the hours that this world-famous scientist would spend on the phone counseling them and others, without any thought of compensation.

Time went by and then, in November 2011, I was shocked to learn that Lloyd had passed away from prostate cancer, which had been discovered in an advanced stage. In January 2012, I was invited by the head of the Cancer Research Institute to attend Old's memorial service at MSKCC.

Top immunologists came from around the world to pay homage. But there was not a single mention of his life-long involvement with what is now called complementary and alternative medicine (CAM), and especially of his pivotal role in the laetrile studies. Some obituaries even left out all reference to his involvement with Helen Coley Nauts and her father's toxins. But his advocacy of CAM in the 1970s set the stage for the formation in the 1990s of the Office of Alternative Medicine (now the National Center for Complementary and Alternative Medicine, NCCAM), and was in my opinion among his greatest contributions.

In June 1999, I had an even more memorable homecoming. Against all expectations, I was invited to deliver a lecture to the MSKCC Department of Surgery. This resulted from my friendship with the chairman of MSKCC's urology department, William R. Fair, MD (1935-2002). Because of his own battle with colon cancer, Bill Fair had developed an intense interest in complementary and alternative medicine (CAM). He reached out to me through mutual acquaintances and we became friends and colleagues in a number of organizations. Through him I also became friends with several high officials of MSKCC, including one member of the Board of Trustees.

This unexpected re-engagement ultimately led to an invitation from MSKCC's Senior Vice President, Thomas J. Fahey III, MD, to take part in an early-morning seminar for the staff, which is called a "Grand Rounds." Over 100 people, many of them young surgeons, attended. The topic I chose to speak about was, and remains, a fairly controversial one, the interaction of antioxidants with chemotherapy.

But Bill Fair was nervous that I might mention the circumstances of my firing. In his letter of invitation, he wrote:

> "*We will have to keep this strictly clinical, with no reference to laetrile or any previous difficulties with Memorial.*"[342]

Bill's motives were good: he knew how entrenched was the opposition to CAM at Memorial, and he didn't want his own efforts to bring yoga in particular to the surgery department to be derailed by a divisive argument about what happened decades before. I, of course, saw things differently. I hoped for a reckoning of what had actually occurred with laetrile, but I bowed to reality, and accepted the chance of speaking to the MSKCC surgeons, deferring vindication for some later date.

It was personally satisfying for me to reappear at MSKCC after more than 20 years, after having been ordered off the premises by armed guards.

However, as I mounted the podium, just after he introduced me, Bill leaned over and whispered in my ear:

> "*Don't say anything about laetrile!*"

Epilogue

The exclusive focus of this book has been on establishing *what* happened at Sloan-Kettering Institute when it evaluated laetrile in the period 1972-1978. I realize, however, that many readers will be left with other questions on their minds. Among these is *why* the leaders of the "cancer establishment" were so adamantly opposed to laetrile and other non-conventional treatments.

I hope to write more extensively on this question in the future. In the meantime, I suggest that the interested reader consult the Fourth Edition of my book, *The Cancer Industry*, which answers that question in reference to eight complementary and alternative (CAM) treatments, including laetrile. Books are available at Amazon.com and other online booksellers.

End Notes

1   Ross, Warren. Are NDA laws unconstitutional? *Medical Marketing & Media*, March 2007, p. 45.
2   http://www.stanford.edu/dept/classics/cgi-bin/web/news/stanford-classics-tops-national-research-council-rankings
3   Lyman, Richard W. Stanford in turmoil. *Sandstone & Tile*. 2011;35:5-14.
4   United States. Congress. Senate. Labor and Public Welfare. *National Cancer Act of 1974: Hearing Before the Subcommittee on Health*, Jan. 30, 1974, p. 282.
5   Saxon, Wolfgang. Gerard Piel, 89, who revived *Scientific American* magazine, dies. *New York Times,* September 7, 2004.
6   Balis ME, Borenfreund E, Brown GB, et al. Aaron Bendich: 1917-1979, *Cancer Res.* 1980;40:493.
7   Bendich A, Borenfreund E, Sternberg SS. Penetration of somatic mammalian cells by sperm. *Science.* 1974;183:857–859.
8   Manfredi G, Thyagarajan D, Papadopoulou LC, Pallotti F, Schon EA. The fate of human sperm-derived mtDNA in somatic cells. *Am J Hum Genet.* 1997;61:953–960. doi:10.1086/514887.
9   Cooper MD. Robert A. Good May 21, 1922–June 13, 2003. J *Immunol.* 2003;171:6318–6319.
10 Schmeck, Harold M., Nixon drive to conquer cancer is unlikely to succeed quickly. *New York Times,* January 27, 1972, p. 15
11 Strickland, Stephen Parks. *Politics, Science, and Dread Disease.* Cambridge, MA: Harvard University Press, 1972, p. 260.
12 Ibid.
13 Schmeck, Harold M., Jr. Op. cit.
14 Patterson, James T. *The Dread Disease: Cancer and Modern American Culture.* Cambridge, MA: Harvard University Press, 1989, p. 248.
15 Bishop, Jerry E. National goal: curing cancer by 1976. *Wall Street Journal*, Aug. 26, 1970, p. 8.
16 Patterson, James T. *The Dread Disease.*
17 Bishop, Jerry E. Op. cit..
18 http://obf.cancer.gov/financial/factbook.htm
19 Oppel, Richard A., Jr. Benno C. Schmidt, financier, is dead at 86, *New York Times*, October 22, 1999.
20 http://www.smokershistory.com/Schmidt.htm
21 Anonymous (David N. Leff). Laetrile flunks new lab tests. *Medical World News*, August 11, 1975, p. 21.
22 Culliton, Barbara J. Laetrile at Sloan-Kettering: The trails of an apricot pit—1973. *Science*, 1973;182:1000-1003.
23 Ibid.
24 Ibid.
25 Reilly HC, Falco E, Myron SA, Philips FS, Stock CC. Sarcoma 180 screening data. *Cancer Res.* 1963;23:1731-1877.
26 Culliton BJ. Op. cit.
27 http://www.cancerresearch.org/about/lloyd-j-old
28 Carswell-Richards EA and Williamson BD. A man of vision and the discovery of tumor necrosis factor. *Cancer Immunity.* 2012;12:4.
29 Wakeman, Robert Peel. *Wakeman Genealogy, 1630-1899.* Meriden,

Connecticut: Journal Pub. 1900, p. 75.

30   http://www.jci.org/articles/view/64110

31   http://www.cancerresearch.org/about/lloyd-j-old/75th-birthday-tribute

32   Old LJ, Clarke DA, Benacerraf. Effect of Bacillus Calmette-Guerin infection on transplanted tumours in the mouse. *Nature.* 1959;184:291–292.

33   Old LJ, Boyse EA. Current enigmas in cancer research. *Harvey Lect.* 1973;67:273–315.

34   http://www.jci.org/articles/view/64110

35   Helen Coley Nauts, letter to the author, March 22, 1991.

36   http://www.cancerresearch.org/about/lloyd-j-old

37   Good RA, Venters H, Page AR, Good TA. Diffuse connective tissue disease in childhood with a special comment on connective tissue diseases in patients with agammaglobulinemia. *J Lancet.* 1961;81:192–204.

38   Maclean LD, Zak SJ, Varco RL, Good RA. The role of the thymus in antibody production; an experimental study of the immune response in thymectomized rabbits. *Transplant Bull.* 1957;4:21–22.

39   Ribatti D. The fundamental contribution of Robert A. Good to the discovery of the crucial role of thymus in mammalian immunity. *Immunology.* 2006;119:291–295.

40   Gupta S, Pahwa R, Siegal FP, Good RA. Rosette formation with mouse erythrocytes. IV. T, B and third population cells in human tonsils. *Clin Exp Immunol.* 1977;28:347–351.

41   Wade, Nicholas. Laetrile at Sloan-Kettering: A question of ambiguity. *Science.* 1977;198:1231-1234.

42   Hixson, Joseph. *The Patchwork Mouse.* Garden City, NY: Doubleday & Co., 1976.

43   Fernandes G, Yunis EJ, Good RA. Influence of diet on survival of mice. *Proc Natl Acad Sci. U.S.A.* 1976;73:1279–1283.

44   Burkitt, Denis. *Don't Forget Fibre in your Diet: To Help Avoid Many of our Commonest Diseases.* Denis London: Martin Dunitz Ltd., 1979.

45   Hixson. Op. cit.

46   Ibid.

47   Summerlin WT, Charlton E, Karasek M. Transplantation of organ cultures of adult human skin. *J Invest Dermatol.* 1970;55:310-316.

48   Meyers, Morton, MD. *Prize Fight: The Race and the Rivalry to be the First in Science.* Palgrave-Macmillan, 2012, p. 55.

49   Stoler, Peter. Toward cancer control. *Time.* March 19, 1973 {cover story}.

50   Hixson. Op. cit.

51   Stansfield, William D. *Death of a Rat: Understandings and Appreciations of Science.* Amherst, NY: Prometheus Books, 2000.

52   Anonymous. Fraud laid to scientist. *Post-Standard,* Syracuse, NY, May 25, 1975, p. 2.

53   Brody, Jane. Inquiry at cancer center finds fraud in research. *New York Times,* May 25, 1974, p. 1.

54   Hixson. Op. cit.

55   Ninnemann JL, Good RA. Allogeneic transplantation of organ cultures without immunosuppression. An evaluation using adult mouse skin. *Transplantation.* 1974;18:1-5.

56   Doughman DJ, Van Horn D, Harris JE, et al. Endothelium of the human organ cultured cornea: an electron microscopic study. *Trans Am Ophthalmol Soc.* 1973;71:304–324; discussion 325–328.

57   Summerlin WT, Miller GE, Harris JE, Good RA. The organ-cultured cornea:

an in vitro study. *Invest Ophthalmol.* 1973;12:176-180.

58   Summerlin WT, Broutbar C, Foanes RB, et al. Acceptance of phenotypically differing cultured skin in man and mice. *Transplant Proc.* 1973;5:707-710.

59   Culliton, Barbara J. Sloan-Kettering affair: a story without a hero. *Science.* 1974;184:644-650.

60   Brody, Jane E. Charge of false research data stirs cancer scientists at Sloan-Kettering. *New York Times,* April 17, 1974.

61   Medawar, Peter. The strange case of the spotted mice. (A review of *The Patchwork Mouse* by Joseph Hixson). *The New York Review of Books.* 1976;23(6):6.

62   Culliton, Barbara J. Op. cit.

63   Hixson. Op. cit., p. 101.

64   Culliton, Barbara J. The Sloan-Kettering affair (II): An uneasy resolution. *Science.* 1974;184:1154-1157.

65   Snow, CP. The *Two Cultures and the Scientific Revolution.* Cambridge, UK: Cambridge University Press, 2013. (Lecture first delivered in 1959).

66   Thomas, Lewis. *The Lives of a Cell.* New York: Viking Press, 1974.

67   http://www.the-scientist.com/?articles.view/ articleNo/32219/title/Alternative-Medicines/flagPost/64986/

68   Anonymous. Cornerstone set in war on cancer. *New York Times,* June 7, 1958, p. 20.

69   Morgan IM, Schlesinger RW, Olitsky PK. Induced resistance of the central nervous system to experimental infection with equine encephalomyelitis virus *J Exp Med.* 1942;76:357–369.

70   Sugiura K. Reminiscence and experience in experimental chemotherapy of cancer. *Med Clin North Am.* 1971;55:667-82.

71   Ibid.

72   Roosevelt, Theodore. *Theodore Roosevelt's Letters to His Children,* Joseph Bucklin Bishop, ed. New York: Charles Scribner's Sons, 1919, pp. 113-114.

73   Anonymous. Jiu-jitsu as in Japan. *New York Times,* Feb. 4, 1906.

74   Ibid.

75   Sugiura K. Reminiscence and experience in experimental chemotherapy of cancer. *Med Clin North Am.* 1971;55:667–682.

76   Anonymous. Jiu-Jitsu as in Japan. *New York Times,* Feb. 4, 1906.

77   Sugiura K. Op. cit.

78   Hutchison, Dorris J. Kanematsu Sugiura 1890-1979 (obituary). *Cancer Res.* 1980;40:2625-2626.

79   Sugiura K. Op. cit.

80   Zantinga AR, Coppes MJ. James Ewing (1866-1943): "The Chief." *Med Pediatr Oncol.* 1993;21:505–510.

81   Hutchison, Dorris J. Op.cit.

82   Sugiura K. The carcinogenicity of certain compounds related to p-dimethylaminoazobenzene. Cancer Res. 1948;8:141–144.

83   Kensler CJ, Sugiura K, Young NF, Halter CR, Rhoads CP.. Partial protection of rats by riboflavin with casein against liver cancer caused by dimethyl-aminoazobenzene. *Science.* 1941;93:308-310.

84   Lal GB. Science. *Alburquerque Journal,* April 1, 1941, p.6.

85   Associated Press. Sugiura dies: Was pioneer. *Reading Eagle,* Oct. 23, 1979, p. 29.

86   Ennis, Thomas W. Dr. Kanematsu Sugiura, 89, dies; A pioneer in cancer chemotherapy. *New York Times,* Oct. 23, 1979.

87   Hata T, Hoshi T, Kanamori K. Mitomycin, a new antibiotic from Streptomyces.

I J Antibiot. 1956;9:141–146.

88   Sugiura K, Failla G. Some effects of radium radiations on white mice. J. Gen. Physiol. 1922;4:423–436.

89   Dodson, Lynne. *A Century of Oncology: A Photographic History of Cancer Research.* Greenwich, CT: Greenwich Press, 1997.

90   Sugiura, Kanematsu. *The Publications of Kanematsu Sugiura: Memorial Edition.* 4 vols. Foreword by C. Chester Stock. New York: Sloan-Kettering Institute, 1965.

91   Shimkin, Michael B. *Contrary to Nature.* DHEW Pub. No. (NIH) 76-720. Bethesda, Md.: National Institutes of Health, 1977:404.

92   Sinclair, Upon. *I, Candidate for Governor: And How I Got Licked.* Berkeley: University of California Press, 1994, p. 109.

93   Cortazzi, Hugh. Loyalty alone is not enough. *Japan Times,* Jan. 18, 2012.

94   http://www.sdbjj.com/bjj_etiquette.php

95   http://tribstar.com/history/x1155671027/Historical-Perspective-A-look-at-the-lives-of-William-Thomas-Burke-and-Charles-Chester-Stock/print

96   Ibid.

97   Martin DS. The role of the surgeon in the prospect of death from cancer. *CA: A Cancer Journal for Clinicians.* 1968;18:264-267.

98   Ibid.

99   Martin, Daniel S. A review of amygdalin-laetrile [mimeographed pamphlet]. New York, 1976.

100   Anonymous (David N. Leff). Laetrile testing: a cover-up that wasn't. *Medical World News,* October 26, 1975.

101   Associated Press (Brian Sullivan). Laetrile swindle. *The Albany Herald,* Albany, Ga., May 4, 1977, p. 8.

102   http://www.cancer.gov/cancertopics/factsheet/NCI/drugdiscovery

103   Windhorst, Dorothy, MD. Executive secretary, Tumor Immunology Contracting Program, National Cancer Institute, letter to Daniel S. Martin, August 7, 1973. Photocopy in *Second Opinion Special Report,* p. 37.

104   Anonymous (David N. Leff). Laetrile testing: a cover-up that wasn't. *Medical World News,* October 26, 1975.

105   Anonymous (David N. Leff). Laetrile flunks new lab tests. *Medical World News,* August 11, 1975, p. 23.

106   Landing BH, Goldin A, Noe HA, et al. Systemic pathological effects of nitrogen mustards, and a comparison of toxicity, chemical structure, and cytotoxic effect, with reference to the chemotherapy of tumors. *Cancer.* 1949;2:1055–1066.

107   Shapiro DM, Gellhorn A. Combinations of chemical compounds in experimental cancer therapy. *Cancer Res.* 1951;11:35–41.

108   Shapiro DM, Warren S. Cancer innervation. *Cancer Res.* 1949;9:707–711.

109   Martin DS, Kligerman MM, Fugmann RA. Radiotherapy and adjuvant combination chemotherapy (6-aminonicotinamide and 6-mercaptopurine). *Cancer Res.* 1958;18:893–896.

110   Shapiro DM, Goldin A. Cancer chemotherapy; analysis of results of different screening techniques with nitrogen-mustard analogues. *Cancer.* 1949;2:100–112.

111   Merluzzi VJ, Savage DM, Souza L, et al. Lysis of spontaneous murine breast tumors by human interleukin 2-stimulated syngeneic T-lymphocytes. *Cancer Res.* 1985;45:203–206.

112   Martin DS. An appraisal of chemotherapy as an adjuvant to surgery for cancer. *Am J Surg.* 1959;97:685–686.

113   Martin, Daniel S. The necessity for combined modalities in cancer therapy. In: Kruse, LC, Reese, JL, and Hart, LK. *Cancer: Pathophysiology, Etiology, and Management: Selected Readings.* St. Louis: Mosby, 1979, p. 248.

114   Martin DS, Hayworth PE, Fugmann RA. Enhanced cures of spontaneous murine mammary tumors with surgery, combination chemotherapy, and immunotherapy. *Cancer Res.* 1970;30:709–716.

115   Comen E, Norton L, Massagué J. Clinical implications of cancer self-seeding. *Nature Reviews Clinical Oncology.* 2011;8:369–77.

116   Hendren, Harriet. Retiree volunteers to help fight hunger in new setting. *Herald-Leader*, Lexington, KY, June 12, 1991, p. 8.

117   Stolfi RL, Martin DS, Fugmann RA. Spontaneous murine mammary adenocarcinoma: model system for evaluation of combined methods of therapy. *Cancer Chemother Rep.* 1971;55:239–251.

118   Daniel S. Martin v. Catholic Medical Center Brooklyn and Queens, Supreme Court of New York, Appellate Division, First Department, Nov. 20, 1973.

119   Ibid.

120   Louise, Kathleen. Historic St. Anthony's hospital to be demolished in 2 months. Nov. 22, 2001. (Retrieved from qchron.com)

121   http://ny.findacase.com/

122   Windhorst, Dorothy. Letter to Daniel S. Martin, MD. August 7, 1973. Reproduced in *Second Opinion Special Report*, p. 37.

123   Anonymous. Ineffective cancer therapy: a guide for the layperson. *J Clin Oncol.* 1983;1:154–163.

124   Martin, Daniel S. Laetrile worthless. *Daily Gazette*, Xenia, OH, June 11, 1977.

125   Zinser, Ben. Medicine and you. *Independent Press-Telegram*, Long Beach, California, Dec. 26, 1977.

126   United Press International. Experts say laetrile useless. *Florence Times-TriCities Daily*, Shoals, Alabama, Feb. 9, 1978, p. 22.

127   Anonymous. Paid notice: deaths. Martin, Daniel S., MD. *New York Times*, July 9, 2005.

128   Wade, Nicholas. Laetrile at Sloan-Kettering: A question of ambiguity. *Science.* 1977;198: 1231-1234.

129   Anonymous (David N. Leff). Laetrile testing: a cover-up that wasn't. *Medical World News*, October 26, 1975.

130   Sloan-Kettering Institute, Laetrile press conference, June 15, 1977. ABC news roll, @ TCR 01:16:25:14 (obtained by Eric Merola).

131   Anonymous. Drug attacks prostate cancer in mouse model by destroying its blood supply. *M.D. Anderson News Release*, June 6, 2006.

132   Melamed MR, Darzynkiewicz Z, Traganos F, Sharpless T. Cytology automation by flow cytometry. *Cancer Res.* 1977;37:2806–2812.

133   http://www.zionchapel.com/obituaries/Myron-Melamed/#!/Obituary

134   Dodson, Jeanne L. Op. cit.

135   http://www.mskcc.org/cancer-care/pathology-consultations

136   Medawar, Peter. The strange case of the spotted mice. A review of *The Patchwork Mouse* by Joseph Hixson. *The New York Review of Books.* 1976;23:6

137   Manner, Harold. *The Death of Cancer.* Chicago: Advanced Century Publishing Corp., 1978.

138   Edson, Lee. Why laetrile won't go away. *New York Times Magazine*, November 27, 1977.

139   Anderson JC, Fugmann RA, Stolfi RL, Martin DS. Metastatic incidence of a spontaneous murine mammary adenocarcinoma. *Cancer Res.* 1974;34:1916–1920.

140   Ibid.

141   Ibid.

142   Stock CC, Martin DS, Sugiura K, et al. Antitumor tests of amygdalin in spontaneous animal tumor systems. *J Surg Oncol.* 1978;10:89–123, p. 91.

143   Tibbetts P. Notes and Discussions: The subjective element in scientific discovery: Popper versus "traditional epistemology." *Dialectica.* 1980;34:155–160.

144   Winsberg E. Models of success versus the success of models: reliability without truth. *Synthese.* 2006;152:1–19.

145   Brown, Tony. *Mathematics Education and Subjectivity: Cultures and Cultural Renewal,* Dordrecht: Springer, 2011.

146   Naples, Michael J. *Effective Frequency.* New York: McGraw Hill, 1979.

147   Connolly JL, Schnitt SJ, Wang HH, Dvorak AM, Dvorak HF. *Principles of Cancer Pathology. In: Holland-Frei Cancer Medicine,* Hamilton, Ontario: BC Decker, 2000, ch. 29.

148   Articles are to be found at aacrjournals.org

149   Harada Y. Pituitary role in the growth of metastasizing MRMT-1 mammary carcinoma in rats. *Cancer Res.* 1976;36:18–22.

150   Yuhas JM, Ullrich RL. Responsiveness of senescent mice to the antitumor properties of Corynebacterium parvum. *Cancer Res.* 1976;36:161–166.

151   Liotta LA, Saidel MG, Kleinerman J. The significance of hematogenous tumor cell clumps in the metastatic process. *Cancer Res.* 1976;36:889–894.

152   Franks LM, Carbonell AW, Hemmings VJ, Riddle PN. Metastasizing tumors from serum-supplemented and serum-free cell lines from a C57BL mouse lung tumor. *Cancer Res.* 1976;36:1049–1055.

153   Dubois JB, Serrou B. Treatment of the mouse Lewis tumor by the association of radiotherapy and immunotherapy with Bacillus Calmette-Guérin. *Cancer Res.* 1976;36:1731–1734.

154   Carmel RJ, Brown JM. The effect of cyclophosphamide and other drugs on the incidence of pulmonary metastases in mice. *Cancer Res.* 1977;37:145–151.

155   Ushio Y, Chernik NL, Shapiro WR, Posner JB. Metastic tumor of the brain: development of an experimental model. *Ann Neurol.* 1977;2:20–29.

156   Mulé JJ, Yang J, Shu S, Rosenberg SA. The anti-tumor efficacy of lymphokine-activated killer cells and recombinant interleukin 2 in vivo: direct correlation between reduction of established metastases and cytolytic activity of lymphokine-activated killer cells. *J Immunol.* 1986;136:3899–3909.

157   Panigrahy D, Edin ML, Lee CR, et al. Epoxyeicosanoids stimulate multiorgan metastasis and tumor dormancy escape in mice. *J Clin Invest.* 2012;122:178–191.

158   O'Dell MR, Huang J-L, Whitney-Miller CL, et al. KrasG12D and p53 mutation cause primary intra-hepatic cholangiocarcinoma. *Cancer Res.* 2012;72:1557–1567.

159   Said N, Sanchez-Carbayo M, Smith SC, Theodorescu D. RhoGDI2 suppresses lung metastasis in mice by reducing tumor versican expression and macrophage infiltration. *J Clin Invest.* 2012;122:1503–1518.

160   Guo L, Fan D, Zhang F, et al. Selection of Brain Metastasis-Initiating Breast Cancer Cells Determined by Growth on Hard Agar. *Am J Pathol.* 2011;178:2357–2366.

161   Lindsay CR, Lawn S, Campbell AD, et al. P-Rex1 is required for efficient melanoblast migration and melanoma metastasis. *Nat Commun.* 2011;2:555.

162   Guo L, Fan D, Zhang F, et al. Selection of brain metastasis-initiating breast cancer cells. *Am J Pathol.* 2011;178:2357–2366.

163   Unemori EN, Ways N, Pitelka DR. Metastasis of murine mammary tumour lines from the mammary gland and ectopic sites. *Br J Cancer*. 1984;49:603–614.

164   Ware JL, DeLong ER. Influence of tumour size on human prostate tumour metastasis in athymic nude mice. *Br J Cancer*. 1985;51:419–423.

165   Anderson JC, Fugmann RA, Stolfi RL, Martin DS. Metastatic incidence of a spontaneous murine mammary adenocarcinoma. *Cancer Res*. 1974;34:1916–1920.

166   Burger AM, Fiebig HH. Preclinical screening for new anticancer agents. In: Figg WD, McLeod HL (Eds.) *Handbook of Anticancer Pharmacokinetics and Pharmacodynamics*. Springer, 2004.

167   Suggitt M, Bibby MC. 50 years of preclinical anticancer drug screening: empirical to target-driven approaches. *Clin Cancer Res*. 2005;11:971–981.

168   Wustrow TP, Katopodis N, Stock CC, Good RA. Prevention of leukemia and the increase of plasma levels of lipid-bound sialic acid by allogeneic bone marrow transplantation in mice. *Cancer Res*. 1985;45:1097–1100.

169   Fugmann RA, Anderson JC, Stolfi RL, Martin DS. Comparison of adjuvant chemotherapeutic activity against primary and metastatic spontaneous murine tumors. *Cancer Res*. 1977;37:496–500.

170   Ibid.

171   Anderson JC, Fugmann RA, Stolfi RL, Martin DS. Metastatic incidence of a spontaneous murine mammary adenocarcinoma. *Cancer Res*. 1974;34:1916–1920.

172   Stock CC, Martin DS, Sugiura K, et al. Antitumor tests of amygdalin in spontaneous animal tumor systems. *J Surg Oncol*. 1978;10:89–123.

173   Ritzi E, Martin DS, Stolfi RL, Spiegelman S. Plasma levels of a viral protein as a diagnostic signal for the presence of tumor : the murine mammary tumor model. *Proc Natl Acad Sci USA*. 1976;73:4190–4194.

174   Martin DS. The scientific basis for adjuvant chemotherapy. *Cancer Treat Rev*. 1981;8:169–189.

175   Kelsen D, Martin DS, Colofiore J, Sawyer R, Coit D. A phase II trial of biochemical modulation using N-phosphonacetyl-L-aspartate, high-dose methotrexate, high-dose 5-fluorouracil, and leucovorin in patients with adenocarcinoma of unknown primary site. *Cancer*. 1992;70:1988–1992.

176   Martin DS. The scientific basis for adjuvant chemotherapy. *Cancer Treat Rev*. 1981;8:169–189.

177   Kelsen D, et al. A phase II trial of biochemical modulation. *Cancer*. 1992;70:1988-1992.

178   Salsburg DS. Use of statistics when examining lifetime studies in rodents to detect carcinogenicity. *J Toxicol Environ Health*. 1977;3:611–628.

179   Manuppello J, Willett C. Longer Rodent Bioassay Fails to Address 2-Year Bioassay's Flaws. *Environ Health Perspect*. 2008;116:A516–A517.

180   Committee for Freedom of Choice in Cancer, Inc. *Anatomy of a Cover-up*, Los Altos, CA, August 1975.

181   Stock CC, Tarnowski GS, Schmid FA, Hutchison DJ, Teller MN. Antitumor tests of amygdalin in transplantable animal tumor systems. *J Surg Oncol*. 1978;10:81–88.

182   Wodinsky I, Swiniarski JK. Antitumor activity of amygdalin MF (NSC-15780) as a single agent and with beta-glucosidase (NSC-128056) on a spectrum of transplantable rodent tumors. *Cancer Chemother Rep*. 1975;59:939–950.

183   Stock CC, et al. Op. cit.

184   Culliton BJ. Sloan-Kettering: the trials of an apricot pit-1973. *Science*.

1973;182:1000–1003.

185   Boyd MR. The NCI In vitro anticancer drug discovery screen. In: *Concept, Implementation, and Operation, 1985-1995. Anticancer Drug Development Guide: Preclinical Screening, Clinical Trials, and Approval.* (Edited by B. Teicher.) Totowa, NJ: Humana Press Inc., 1995.

186   http://www.ncbi.nlm.nih.gov/books/NBK20822/

187   Martin DS, Hayworth P, Fugmann RA, English R, McNeill HW. Combination therapy with cyclophosphamide and zymosan on a spontaneous mammary cancer in mice. *Cancer Res.* 1964;24:652–654.

188   Chihara G, Hamuro J, Maeda Y, Arai Y, Fukuoka F. Fractionation and purification of the polysaccharides with marked antitumor activity, especially lentinan, from Lentinus edodes (Berk.) Sing. (an edible mushroom). *Cancer Res.* 1970;30:2776–2781.

189   Culliton. Op. cit.

190   Anderson JC, Fugmann RA, Stolfi RL, Martin DS. Metastatic incidence of a spontaneous murine mammary adenocarcinoma. *Cancer Res.* 1974;34:1916–1920.

191   Culliton. Op. cit.

192   Nelson, Harry. Laetrile. A typewritten manuscript preserved at the University of California San Francisco library and retrieved from: http://legacy.library.ucsf.edu/tid/tuy3aa00/pdf

193   Aggarwal BB, Shishodia S, Takada Y, et al. Curcumin suppresses the paclitaxel-induced nuclear factor-kappaB pathway in breast cancer cells and inhibits lung metastasis of human breast cancer in nude mice. *Clin Cancer Res.* 2005;11:7490–7498.

194   Furth, J, Siebold HR, Rathbone RR. Experimental studies on lymphomatosis of mice. *Am J Cancer.* 1933;19:521-590.

195   Furth J. The creation of the AKR Strain, whose DNA contains the genome of a leukemia virus. In: Morse 3rd HC (Ed.). *Origins of Inbred Mice.* New York: Academic Press, 1978.

196   Kassel RL, Old LJ, Carswell EA, Fiore NC, Hardy WD Jr. Serum-mediated leukemia cell destruction in AKR mice. *J Exp Med.* 1973;138:925–938.

197   Sugiura, K. Memo (on Sloan-Kettering letterhead). Dated May 17, 1975. Photocopied and republished in *Second Opinion Special Report: Laetrile at Sloan-Kettering,* p. 33.

198   Quoted in *Second Opinion Special Report: Laetrile at Sloan-Kettering,* Bronx, New York: Second Opinion, 1977, p. 21.

199   Sugiura, Kanematsu. Memo of July 25, 1975, reprinted in *Second Opinion Special Report: Laetrile at Sloan-Kettering,* 1977, p. 32.

200   Kassel RL, Old LJ, Carswell EA, et al. Serum-mediated leukemia cell destruction in AKR mice. *J Exper Med.* 1973;138:925–939.

201   Graff S, Kassel R, Kastner O. Interferon. *Trans N Y Acad Sci.* 1970;32:545–556.

202   Kassel R, Hardy W, Day NK. Complement in cancer. In: *Biological Amplification Systems in Immunology.* Day NK and Good RA, eds. New York: Plenum, 1977:277-294 (particularly pp. 280-281).

203   Stock CC, Martin DS, Sugiura K, et al. Antitumor tests of amygdalin in spontaneous animal tumor systems. *J Surg Oncol.* 1978;10:89–123.

204   Hayashi I, Ohotsuki M, Suzuki I, Watanabe T. Effects of oral administration of Echinacea purpurea (American herb) on incidence of spontaneous leukemia caused by recombinant leukemia viruses in AKR/J mice. *Japan J Clin Immunol.* 2001;24;10-20.

205   Ibid.

206   Sugiura K, Hitchings GH, Cavalieri LF, Stock CC. The Effect of 8-Azaguanine on the growth of carcinoma, sarcoma, etc. *Cancer Res.* 1950;10:178–185.

207   Sugiura K. Experimental production of carcinoma in mice with cigarette smoke tar. *Gann.* 1956;47:243–244.

208   Ibid.

209   Brody, Jane. Four cancer centers find no proof of therapy value in illegal drug. *New York Times,* July 21, 1975, p.1.

210   Quoted in *Second Opinion Special Report: Laetrile at Sloan-Kettering*, Bronx, New York: Second Opinion, 1977.

211   Culliton BJ. Sloan-Kettering: the trials of an apricot pit-1973. *Science.* 1973;182:1000–1003.

212   Ibid.

213   Villavicencio JL, Merrill DM, Rich NM. The military medical school of Mexico: a tradition of excellence. *World J Surg.* 2005;29 Suppl 1:S99–104.

214   Sloan-Kettering Institute. *Minutes, Meeting on Amygdalin.* New York, July 10, 1973.

215   Ibid.

216   Madison [Wisconsin] *Capital Times*, November 3, 1973.

217   Dean Burk to Ralph W. Moss. Personal communication, Dec. 13, 1977 (cited in *The Cancer Industry*).

218   Schloen, Lloyd H. Notes from First Annual Convention of the International Association of Cancer Victims and Friends, Inc. New York, April 15, 1973. Memorandum prepared for the MSKCC administration.

219   Memorial Sloan-Kettering Cancer Center, Department of Public Affairs. *Official Laetrile Statement*, Fall, 1973.

220   Culliton. Op. cit.

221   Ibid.

222   Ibid.

223   McGrady, Patrick M. The American Cancer Society means well, but the Janker Clinic means better. *Esquire*, April 1976.

224   Brody JE and Holleb AI. *You Can Fight Cancer and Win.* New York: McGraw Hill, 1974.

225   Cited in McGrady, Jr. Op. cit.

226   MSKCC *Center News,* January, 1975.

227   Anonymous. The Nation. *Los Angeles Times*, Jan. 10, 1974, p. A2.

228   Kotulak, Ronald. Study finds controversial drug ineffective as cure for cancer. *Chicago Tribune,* Jan. 10, 1974, p. A11.

229   Kuznetsky, Dan. PR and the art of misdirection, April 26, 2013. Retrieved December 3, 2013 from: http://www.zdnet.com/pr-and-the-art-of-misdirection-7000014576/

230   Anonymous. Rochester (Minn.) *Post Bulletin.* January 21, 1974.

231   Anonymous. FDA chief raps cancer drug use. *Charleston Daily Mail*, March 25, 1974, p.11A [Syndication of *New York Daily News* article].

232   Anonymous. In the news this morning. *Oneonta Star,* March 25, 1974, p.1.

233   Anonymous. FDA chief raps cancer drug use. *Charleston Daily Mail*, March 25, 1974, p.11A [syndicated from *New York Daily News*].

234   Carpenter, Daniel. *Reputation and Power: Organizational Image and Pharmaceutical Regulation at the FDA.* Princeton: Princeton University Press, 2010, p. 423.

235   Associated Press. Cancer specialists give new drug failing grade. *Morning News*, Florence, NC, March 25, 1974, p. 5.

236   Culliton. Op. cit.

237   Ibid.
238   Moertel CG, Fleming TR, Rubin J, et al. A clinical trial of amygdalin (Laetrile) in the treatment of human cancer. *N Engl J Med.* 1982;306:201-206.
239   Culliton. Op. cit.
240   Griffin G. Edward. *World Without Cancer,* Westlake Village, CA: American Media,1975, p. 464.
241   Minutes, FDA meeting on laetrile, July 1974.
242   Carpenter, Daniel. Op. cit.
243   Jacobs, Paul. Mayo cancer researcher is 'Dr. Debunker.' *Los Angeles Times,* Jan. 29, 1982, p. B15.
244   Case DC, Hansen JA, Corrales E, et al. Comparison of multiple in vivo and in vitro parameters in untreated patients with Hodgkin's disease. *Cancer.* 1976;38:1807–1815.
245   Case DC Jr, Hansen JA, Corrales E, et al. Depressed in vitro lymphocyte responses to PHA in patients with Hodgkin disease in continuous long remissions. *Blood.* 1977;49:771–778.
246   Schulof RS, Bockman RS, Garofalo JA, et al. Multivariate analysis of T-cell functional defects and circulating serum factors in Hodgkin's disease. *Cancer.* 1981;48:964–973.
247   Anonymous. Treatment of cancer with laetriles; a report by the Cancer Commission of the California Medical Association. *Calif Med.* 1953;78:320-326.
248   Anonymous. *Evening Tribune,* San Diego, Calif. April 2,1975.
249   Culliton. Op. cit.
250   Interlandi, Jeneen. An unwelcome discovery. *New York Times Magazine,* October 22, 2006.
251   Associated Press. Laetrile 'useless as cancer cure.' *Oakland Tribune,* April 3, 1975, p. 17.
252   Holles, Everett R. U.S. indicts 19 in plot to smuggle illegal cancer drug. *New York Times,* May 26, 1975, *Week in Review,* p. 81. *Note:* In the archives of *NYTimes.com* this article is incorrectly dated May 26, 1976. But the identical story from the *New York Times Service* appeared in other American newspapers on May 26, 1975. These included "Illegal cancer-drug smuggling probed," St. Petersburg (Fla.) *Times,* May 27, 1975, p. 6-A and "Smugglers make bundle over cancer," The Bangor (Me.) *Daily News,* May 16, 1975, p. 22.
253   Holles, Everett R. Birch Society members tied to smuggling of illegal drug. *New York Times,* June 1, 1976, p.18.
254   Brody. Op. cit.
255   Sugiura K. Tests of compounds against various mouse tumors. *Cancer Res.* 1958;18:46.
256   Sugiura K. Reminiscence and experience in experimental chemotherapy of cancer. *Med Clin North Am.* 1971;55:667-682. (CD8F1 is mentioned there).
257   Anonymous (David N. Leff). Laetrile flunks new lab tests. *Medical World News,* Aug. 11, 1975, p. 21-23.
258   Stock, C. Chester. A second and low opinions of *Second Opinion's Special Report: Laetrile at Sloan-Kettering.* New York: Sloan-Kettering Institute, Nov. 21, 1977.
259   Whyte, William H. *The Organization Man.* New York: Simon & Schuster, 1956.
260   Rosen GM, Shorr RI: Laetrile: end play around the FDA. A review of legal developments. *Ann Intern Med.* 1979:90:418-423.
261   Anonymous. FDA chief raps cancer drug use. *Charleston Daily Mail,* March 25, 1974, p.11A [Syndication of the *New York Daily News*].

262 Krebs, Ernst T., et al. Committee for Freedom of Choice in Cancer, Inc. *Anatomy of a Cover-up,* August, 1975 (contains photocopy of Old's letter).

263 Associated Press (Brian Sullivan). Controversial drug laetrile tested by Sloan-Kettering. *Herald Bulletin,* Anderson, Indiana, Nov. 24, 1975.

264 Associated Press. Blind study to be made of drug laetrile. *Journal,* Sarasota, Fla., Nov. 21, 1975, p. 31.

265 Associated Press. Cancer center plans new laetrile experiments. *The Press-Courier,* Oxnard, Calif., Nov. 24, 1975, p. 9. (See also: Laetrile testing: a cover-up that wasn't. *Medical World News,* October 26, 1975.)

266 Ibid.

267 Carswell-Richards EA and Williamson BD. A man of vision and the discovery of tumor necrosis factor. *Cancer Immunity* 2012;12:4.

268 Anderson JC, Fugmann RA, Stolfi RL, Martin DS. Metastatic incidence of a spontaneous murine mammary adenocarcinoma. *Cancer Res.* 1974;34:1916–1920.

269 Anonymous (David N. Leff). Laetrile flunks new lab tests. *Medical World News,* August 11, 1975, p. 21-23.

270 Ibid.

271 Ibid.

272 Sugiura K, Schmid FA, Schmid MM. Antitumor activity of cytoxan. *Cancer Res.* 1961;21:1412–1420.

273 Jackall, Robert. *Moral Mazes.* Oxford: Oxford University Press, 2009.

274 Passwater, Richard A. *Cancer and its Nutritional Therapies.* New Canaan, CT: Keats, 1978, p. 163.

275 *Second Opinion Special Report: Laetrile at Sloan-Kettering.* Bronx, NY, 1977.

276 Ibid.

277 Wade, Nicholas. Laetrile at Sloan-Kettering: A question of ambiguity. *Science.* 1977;198:1231-1234.

278 Stock CC, Martin DS, Sugiura K, et al. Antitumor tests of amygdalin in spontaneous animal tumor systems. *J Surg Oncol.* 1978;10:89–123.

279 Anonymous (David N. Leff). Laetrile testing: a cover-up that wasn't. *Medical World News,* October 6, 1975, p. 21–23.

280 Stock, C. Chester. Letter to Ruth Fugmann, PhD, dated July 13, 1973, quoted verbatim in the *Second Opinion Special Report,* p. 22.

281 *Second Opinion Special Report: Laetrile at Sloan-Kettering,* Bronx, New York, 1977, p. 22-23.

282 Anderson JC, Fugmann RA, Stolfi RL, Martin DS. Metastatic incidence of a spontaneous murine mammary adenocarcinoma. Cancer Res. 1974;34:1916–1920.

283 Anonymous (David N. Leff). Laetrile flunks new lab tests. *Medical World News,* August 11, 1975, p. 21.

284 Associated Press, Blind study to be made of drug laetrile. *Journal,* Sarasota, Fla., Nov. 21, 1975, p. 31.

285 Anonymous (David N. Leff). Laetrile testing: a cover-up that wasn't. *Medical World News,* October 26, 1975.

286 Anonymous. Laetrile no miracle cure. Press-Republican, Pittsburgh, PA, August 19, 1977.

287 Anonymous. *Second Opinion.* Bronx, New York, 1976;1:1:4.

288 Holden, Constance. Laetrile: "quack" cancer remedy still brings hope to sufferers. *Science.* September 10, 1976:982-985.

289 *Second Opinion Special Report: Laetrile at Sloan-Kettering,* Bronx, New York: Second Opinion, 1977, p. 26.

290   Schmid FA, Hutchison DJ, Otter GM, Stock CC. Deveopment of resistance to combinations of six antimetabolites in mice with L1210 leukemia. *Cancer Treat Rep.* 1976;60:23–27.

291   http://lancasteronline.com/obituaries/local/519722_Glenys-M--Otter.html

292   Schmid FA, Hutchison DJ, Otter GM, Stock CC. Op. cit.

293   http://www.aalas.org/pdf/Caring_for_Animals_Sheets.pdf

294   Ebino KY. Studies on coprophagy in experimental animals. *Jikken Dobutsu.* 1993;42:1–9.

295   Sukemori S, Kurosawa A, Ikeda S, Kurihara Y. Investigation on the growth of coprophagy-prevented rats with supplemented vitamin B12. *J Anim Physiol Anim Nutr (Berl).* 2006;90:402–406.

296   Barnes RH, Fiala G, McGehee B, Brown A. Prevention of coprophagy in the rat. *J Nutr.* 1957;63:489-98.

297   Ibid.

298   Ge BY, Chen HX, Han FM, Chen Y. Identification of amygdalin and its major metabolites in rat urine by LC-MS/MS. *J Chromatogr B Analyt Technol Biomed Life Sci.* 2007;857:281–286.

299   Barnes RH, Fiala G, et al. Op cit.

300   Ibid.

301   Ge BY, Chen HX, Han FM, Chen Y. Identification of amygdalin and its major metabolites in rat urine by LC-MS/MS. *J Chromatogr B Analyt Technol Biomed Life Sci.* 2007;857:281–286.

302   McGraw-Hill. *Modern Healthcare*, vol. 4, 1975, p. 208 mentions White's MSKCC appointment.

303   Brink, Bob. Laetrile: cure-all vitamin? *Palm Beach (Fla.) Post,* June 2, 1976, p. B1.

304   Palast, Greg. *The Best Democracy Money Can Buy.* London: Constable Ltd., 2003.

305   *Second Opinion,* June 1977, p. 3.

306   Martin, Daniel S. Laetrile: 'A Fraud'. *The New York Times,* op-ed, June 3, 1977, p. A23.

307   Anonymous (David N. Leff). Laetrile testing: a cover-up that wasn't. *Medical World News,* October 26, 1975.

308   Zimmermann, Caroline A. *Laetrile: Hope—or Hoax?* New York: Zebra Books, 1977, p. 127.

309   NBC News footage on MSKCC laetrile press conference, 1:19:50;14 to 1:20:15;06. Filmed June 15, 1977. Obtained by Eric Merola, November 2012.

310   Anonymous. Medicine: victories for laetrile's lobbies. *Time,* May 23, 1977.

311   Wade, Nicholas. Laetrile at Sloan-Kettering: A question of ambiguity. *Science.* 1977;198:1231-1234.

312   Edson, Lee. Op. cit.

313   Lewis Thomas, MD. A Statement Concerning Laetrile. United States Congress, Senate Committee on Human Resources, Subcommittee on Health and Scientific Research. *Banning of the drug laetrile from interstate commerce by FDA.* July 12, 1977, pp. 56-61. Reprint from the University of Michigan Library.

314   *Second Opinion Special Report: Laetrile at Sloan-Kettering,* Bronx, New York, 1977, p. 13.

315   Thomas L, Aleu F, Bitensky MW, Davidson M, Gesner B. Studies of PPLO Infection II. the Neurotoxin of Mycoplasma Neurolyticum. *J Exp Med.* 1966;124:1067–1082.

316   Aleu F, Thomas L. Studies of PPLO infection. 3. Electron microscopic study

of brain lesions caused by Mycoplasma neurolyticum toxin. J Exp Med. 1966;124:1083–1088.

317 Rule, Sheila. Cancer aide out in laetrile dispute. *New York Times,* Nov. 24, 1977.

318 Ibid.

319 Ibid.

320 Stock, CC to Rep. John T. Kelsey, dated April 28, 1978. Letter in the Kelsey Archives of the University of Michigan Library. Obtained from librarian Amanda Kaufmann in January 2013.

321 Pressman, Gabe. Television program on laetrile, in a series on cancer. *WNEW-TV,* May 16, 1979.

322 Boffey, PM. Dr. Marks' crusade; shaking up Sloan-Kettering for a new assault on cancer. *New York Times Magazine,* April 26, 1987.

323 Saxon, Wolfgang. Robert A. Good, founder of modern immunology, dies. *New York Times,* June 18, 2003.

324 Shapiro DM, Fugmann RA. A role for chemotherapy as an adjunct to surgery. *Cancer Res.* 1957;17:1098–1101.

325 Martin DS, Fugmann RA. Clinical Implications of the interrelationship of tumor size and chemotherapeutic response. *Ann Surg.* 1960;151:97–100.

326 Martin DS, Hayworth P, Fugmann RA, English R, McNeill HW. Combination therapy with cyclophosphamide and zymosan on a spontaneous mammary cancer in mice. *Cancer Res.* 1964;24:652–654.

327 Martin DS, Hayworth PE, Fugmann RA. Enhanced cures of spontaneous murine mammary tumors with surgery, combination chemotherapy, and immunotherapy. *Cancer Res.* 1970;30:709–716.

328 Martin DS, Fugmann RA, Stolfi RL, Hayworth PE. Solid tumor animal-model therapeutically predictive for human breast cancer. *Cancer Chemotherapy Reports* Part 2. Supplement. 1975;5:89-109.

329 Wade, Nicholas. Laetrile at Sloan-Kettering: A question of ambiguity. *Science.* 1977;198:1231-1234.

330 Ibid.

331 Smith, Richard D. Sloan-Kettering retracts erroneous claim for laetrile tests. *The New York Academy of Sciences News Release,* Dec. 12, 1977.

332 Altman, Lawrence K. Laetrile study data faced by challenge. *New York Times,* Dec. 13, 1977, p. 35.

333 Ibid.

334 Ibid.

335 Ibid.

336 Strange K. Authorship: why not just toss a coin? *Am J Physiol Cell Physiol.* 2008;295:C567–C575.

337 Martin DS, Spriggs D, Koutcher JA. A concomitant ATP-depleting strategy markedly enhances anticancer agent activity. *Apoptosis.* 2001;6:125–131.

338 Stock CC, Martin DS, Sugiura K, et al. Antitumor tests of amygdalin in spontaneous animal tumor systems. *J Surg Oncol.* 1978;10:89–123.

339 Anonymous. Henry Rothblatt, 69, defender of 4 Watergate burglars, dies. *Los Angeles Times,* Sept. 08, 1985.

340 Scheffler Phil, producer. "The establishment vs. Dr. Burton." *60 Minutes,* CBS News, May 18, 1980.

341 Wade, Nicholas. Laetrile at Sloan-Kettering: A question of ambiguity. *Science.* 1977;198:1231-1234.

342 Fair, William. Letter to Ralph W. Moss, May 12, 1999.

Manufactured by Amazon.ca
Acheson, AB

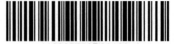

12985759R00133